REHABILITATION MEDICINE

Edited by **Chong-Tae Kim**

Rehabilitation Medicine
Edited by Chong-Tae Kim

Published by InTech

Janeza Trdine 9, 51000 Rijeka, Croatia

Publishing Process Manager Martina Blecic

Technical Editor Teodora Smiljanic

Cover Designer InTech Design Team

Additional hard copies can be obtained from orders@intechopen.com

Rehabilitation Medicine, Edited by Chong-Tae Kim
p. cm.
ISBN 978-953-51-0683-8

For EU product safety concerns:
IN TECH d.o.o., Prolaz Marije Krucifikse Kozulić 3, 51000 Rijeka, Croatia,
info@intechopen.com or visit our website at intechopen.com.

Meet the editor

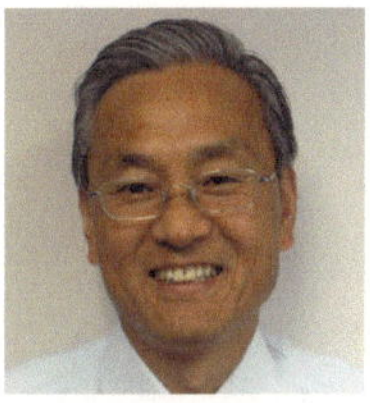

Dr Chong Tae Kim received the both M.D. and Ph. D. degrees from Yonsei University, Seoul, Korea, in 1982 and 1997, respectively. He completed the physical medicine and rehabilitation residency at Yonsei University Hospital, Seoul, Korea from 1986 to 1989 and at Brody Medical School of East Carolina University, Greenville, North Carolina from 1997 to 2001. From 1994 to 1997, he was a research fellow in bioelectricity at Kessler Institute of Rehabilitation, West Orange, New Jersey. Since 2001, he has been an attending physician at the division of pediatric rehabilitation medicine at the Children's Hospital of Philadelphia. His interests are neuro-rehabilitation of pediatric stroke, spinal cord injury, traumatic brain injury, brain tumor, and cerebral palsy.

Contents

Preface IX

Chapter 1 **Diabetic Foot Ulceration and Amputation 1**
Stephanie Burns and Yih-Kuen Jan

Chapter 2 **Stroke Rehabilitation 21**
Chong Tae Kim

Chapter 3 **Myotonometric Measurement of Muscular Properties of Hemiparetic Arms in Stroke Patients 37**
Li-Ling Chuang, Ching-Yi Wu and Keh-Chung Lin

Chapter 4 **Validity and Reliability of a Hand-Held Dynamometer for Dynamic Muscle Strength Assessment 53**
Lan Le-Ngoc and Jessica Janssen

Chapter 5 **Functional Recovery and Muscle Properties After Stroke: A Preliminary Longitudinal Study 67**
Astrid Horstman, Arnold de Haan, Manin Konijnenbelt, Thomas Janssen and Karin Gerrits

Chapter 6 **The Hierarchical Status of Mobility Disability Predicts Future IADL Disability: A Longitudinal Study on Ageing in Taiwan 85**
Hui-Ya Chen, Chih-Jung Yeh, Ching-Yi Wang, Hui-Shen Lin and Meng-Chih Lee

Preface

Rehabilitation medicine is the final care path to improve quality of life for those who sustain impairment, disability, or handicap after illness. Remarkable development and improvement of diagnostic as well as therapeutic skills in recent times have contributed to increasing survival rates. Consequently it also increases demand for rehabilitation for survivors. For rehabilitation professionals, this text will provide current concepts, practical skills, and further research issues in various areas. The contributors of this text not only describe current knowledge, but also stimulate readers to continue developing better rehabilitation skills. This text is not sufficient to cover every rehabilitation issue in one volume. However, we hope the readers will build up more knowledge upon this first edition.

Dr. Chong-Tae Kim
Department of Rehabilitation and Physical Medicine,
University of Pennsylvania, School of Medicine,
USA

1

Diabetic Foot Ulceration and Amputation

Stephanie Burns[1] and Yih-Kuen Jan[2]
[1]*Veterans Affairs Medical Center, Department of Physical Therapy,*
[2]*University of Oklahoma Health Sciences Center, Department of Rehabilitation Sciences, Oklahoma City, Oklahoma, USA*

1. Introduction

The number of people with diabetes mellitus (DM) has been conservatively estimated to approximately double by 2030 to a worldwide prevalence of 4.4% at which time 366 million people will have diabetes (Wild et al., 2004). As the number of people with DM rises, so too will the burden of diabetic foot disease, particularly since the factors contributing to ulcer formation such as peripheral neuropathy and vascular disease are already present in 10% of people at the time of diagnosis (Boulton et al., 2005). The risk of an individual with DM developing a foot ulcer some time in his or her lifetime could be as high as 15% and foot ulcers are found in 12% to 25% of diabetics (Singh et al., 2005; Brem et al., 2006). Results from population and community based studies in the UK have shown a 1.3-4.8% prevalence rate of foot ulcers in persons with type 2 DM (Boulton et al., 2005). The annual incidence of foot ulceration is more than 2% among all persons with diabetes and 5% to 7.6% among diabetics with peripheral neuropathy (Abbott et al., 2002; Boulton et al., 2004).

The prevalence of diabetes-related complications such as peripheral neuropathy and foot disease will continue to increase in countries such as the United States not only as the prevalence of the disease increases but as longevity of the population with DM improves. Among people with DM, lower extremity disease is the most common source of complications and hospitalization (Boyko et al.). Ghanassia et al (2008) reported a diabetic foot ulcer recurrence rate of 60.9% and an amputation rate of 43.8% in a study of 89 hospitalized subjects (Ghanassia et al., 2008). Almost 50% of nontraumatic lower extremity amputations worldwide occur in people with DM (Global Lower Extremity Amputation Study, 2000). Amputations from complications related to DM place an individual at risk for additional amputation and have a 5 year mortality rate of 39% to 68% (Morris et al., 1998). People with diabetic foot ulcers have a lower health-related quality of life than the general population and diabetics without foot ulcers as well (Ribu et al., 2007).

2. Pathophysiology of diabetic foot ulceration

The pathogenesis of diabetic foot ulceration is multifactorial and the result of a complex interplay of a number of elements including peripheral neuropathy, structural deformities, elevated plantar pressures, limited joint mobility, vascular disease, and various extrinsic sources of trauma such as ill fitting shoe wear or foreign objects in shoes. The peripheral neuropathy that occurs in DM is truly a "poly"neuropathy in that sensory, motor and autonomic fibers and function are all adversely affected. It is the sequelae of these neural dysfunctions in conjunction with extrinsic factors that produce the physiologic and structural changes that lead to ulceration. The most common causal pathway to diabetic foot ulceration involves the confluence of loss of sensation resulting in failure to detect repetitive pressure or trauma and abnormal foot structure or deformity producing sites of abnormally high pressure, usually over areas of bony prominence (Mueller et al., 1990; Brem et al., 2006; Chao and Cheing, 2009; O'Loughlin et al., 2010). Diabetic peripheral polyneuropathy is the central component as it can induce changes in foot structure and produce dryness of the skin which can lead to callus formation (van Schie, 2006; O'Loughlin et al., 2010). Callosities form on areas of elevated pressure on the plantar aspect of the foot in response to pressure amplified by restricted joint motion of the ankle and foot which is applied to dry, poorly lubricated skin resulting from autonomic dysfunction (Young et al., 1992). Loss of protective sensation permits continuation of repetitive pressure that goes undetected causing calluses to thicken into sources of tissue trauma then hemorrhage and ulcerate underneath (Murray et al., 1996). Veves et al. (1992) first demonstrated the relationship between high plantar pressures and diabetic foot ulceration in a prospective study in 1992. The relative risk of developing an ulcer in an area of high plantar pressure is 4.7 and that risk more than doubles to 11.0 at the site of a callus (Murray et al., 1996).

2.1 Types of diabetic foot ulcers

Diabetic foot ulcers are classified as one of 3 types based on their primary etiologies and clinical characteristics: neuropathic, neuroischemic, and ischemic. This classification is a reflection of the physiological systems adversely impacted by the chronic hyperglycemia of the disease. Hyperglycemia induces alterations in multiple metabolic pathways resulting in structural and functional changes in the microvasculature of local tissue and the peripheral nerves in cases of peripheral neuropathy (Chao and Cheing, 2009). Neuropathic ulcers appear in the absence of protective sensation as a result of peripheral sensory neuropathy but without evidence of macrovascular disease. The presence of co-morbidity, deep foot infection, and plantar or metatarsal head ulcer location have been shown to be related to minor and major amputation risk in diabetic patients without ischemia (Gershater et al., 2009). They are typically found on the plantar surfaces of the feet and make up about 40% of all diabetic foot ulcers.

Diabetic foot ulcers are considered vascular or ischemic in origin when they occur in the absence of palpable pedal pulses (posterior tibial and dorsalis pedis arteries) in conjunction with ankle brachial indices (ABIs) of less than 0.9. Infection is coincident with ischemia in 50% of patients with this type of diabetic foot ulcer (Dinh et al.; Prompers et al., 2007). This type of ulcer comprises about 10% of all diabetic foot ulcerations. As their name implies, neuroischemic ulcers share features common to both ischemic and neuropathic ulcers in that they occur in the absence of protective sensation and palpable pedal pulses. They make up the final 40% of diabetic foot ulcers. Probability of major amputation in diabetic patients with ischemic/neuroischemic ulcers has been related to the extent of peripheral vascular disease, presence of co-morbidity, multiple ulcerations and tissue loss (Gershater et al., 2009). Peripheral vascular disease is the most important factor related to outcome in these types of diabetic foot ulcers (Boulton et al., 2005; Gershater et al., 2009).

2.2 Diabetic polyneuropathy and ulceration

Nearly 50% of all people with DM have diabetic polyneuropathy making it one of the most common long-term complications of the disease with chronic, symmetrical, sensorimotor polyneuropathy being the most typical type (Tesfaye et al., 2010). Persons with DM and signs of peripheral neuropathy have been shown to be 4 times as likely to have plantar ulcerations as those without neuropathy (Frykberg et al., 1998). Presence of peripheral neuropathy induces a number of pathologic changes in the diabetic foot that then interact to increase susceptibility to ulceration. Sensory neuropathy can affect perception of pain, pressure, touch, temperature, and proprioception. Loss of protective sensation prevents detection of levels of injurious trauma to tissue and stimuli that would ordinarily trigger a protective response such as ill fitting footwear or a foreign object in a shoe go unperceived, often until extensive destruction has occurred. Loss of sensation has been shown to be associated with diabetic foot ulceration in a number of studies (Boyko et al., 1999; Reiber et al., 1999). Results of a prospective multicenter study point to sensory neuropathy as the most frequent component in the causal sequence to diabetic foot ulceration (Reiber et al., 1999). Proprioceptive loss leads to instability and changes in gait that can increase the potential for traumatic injury.

As polyneuropathy progresses, motor fibers are affected resulting in weakness and atrophy of the distal leg and intrinsic foot muscles (Andreassen et al., 2006). Motor neuropathy can lead to foot deformities such as claw or hammertoes, prominent metatarsal heads, or hallux valgus. Prevalence of clawing or hammering toes in persons with DM has been reported to be 32 to 46% (Holewski et al., 1989; Smith et al., 1997). Hammer toe is an important predictor of plantar pressure (Mueller et al., 2003) and claw/hammer toe deformity is associated with elevated plantar pressures at the MTHs (Bus et al., 2005). Intrinsic foot muscle weakness has long been thought to be a proximate cause of deformity in the diabetic foot (Reiber et al., 1999). The intrinsic muscles of the foot ordinarily function to balance the pull of the extrinsic flexors and extensors at the interphalangeal joints by flexing the MTP joints while extending the interphalangeal joints. Weakness of the intrinsic muscles leads to loss of this stabilizing function and ultimately hyperextension of the MTP joints and clawing of the toes. Fat pads underlying the metatarsal heads, embedded in the flexor tendons and originating from the plantar ligaments attached to the proximal phalanges, tend to migrate distally when the toes claw resulting in removal of the soft tissue cushion beneath the metatarsal heads. The prominent metatarsal heads are now exposed to abnormally high plantar pressures during walking as plantar tissue thickness has been shown to be related to peak plantar pressures (Abouaesha et al., 2001). Findings of two recent studies have raised questions about the causal relationship between muscle atrophy and deformity noting that intrinsic muscle atrophy was present before clinical peripheral neuropathy could be detected and finding no significant difference in degree of intrinsic foot muscle atrophy between matched subjects with and without claw toe deformity (Greenman et al., 2005; Bus et al., 2009).

Concomitant damage to the sympathetic fibers in peripheral neuropathy results in sudomotor dysfunction that can trigger a cascade of untoward effects in the foot beginning with atrophy of the sweat glands and progressing through anhidrosis, drying of the skin, fissuring and callus formation (Vinik et al., 2003). Excessive drying has been associated with foot ulceration (Tentolouris et al., 2009). Foot temperature increases in parallel with a reduction in sweating and this may predispose to infection (Sun et al., 2008; O'Loughlin et al., 2010). Tentolouris et al. (2009) found sudomotor dysfunction was associated with an almost 15 times greater risk of foot ulceration and similarly Sun et al. (2008) reported the risk of plantar ulceration occurrence was 13.4 times greater in a patient group with the most sudomotor dysfunction over a 4 year follow-up period.

2.3 Biomechanical factors and ulceration

Limited motion at the ankle or limited joint mobility has been associated with increased peak forefoot pressures and risk of ulceration and re-ulceration (Delbridge et al., 1988). The exact pathogenesis of limited joint mobility in DM is unclear but it is thought to be due to progressive stiffening of the collagen-containing tissues ultimately resulting in thickening of the skin with loss of joint motion (Zimny et al., 2004). Giacomozzi and colleagues demonstrated reduced ankle mobility in patients with DM with and without peripheral neuropathy suggesting another mechanism is responsible for alterations in foot-ankle biomechanics (Giacomozzi et al.). Abnormal thicknesses of plantar fascia and Achilles tendon have been measured (D'Ambrogi et al., 2005; Salsich et al., 2005).

Alterations in biomechanical properties of the diabetic foot have been proven to cause increased plantar foot pressure, which may lead to the development of diabetic foot ulcers (Mueller et al., 2003). Diabetes is associated with the formation of glucose-mediated intermolecular cross-links (i.e. advanced glycation end-products, AGE). Accumulations of AGEs increase stiffness of the cartilages, muscles, tendons, ligaments, and skin (Brownlee et al., 1988). A stiffer plantar soft tissue reduces the shock-absorbing mechanism of the ankle-foot complex and may make the diabetic foot more vulnerable to repetitive stress during walking (Landsman et al., 1995).

The hallux has been identified as the most common site of diabetic foot ulceration, accounting for 20% to 30% of diabetic foot ulcers in a study of 360 patients and comprising 22% of the ulcers seen in another research group's clinic (Armstrong et al., 1998; Nube et al., 2006). Several risk factors have been associated with ulceration of the hallux. Decreased dorsiflexion at the first metatarsophalangeal joint, neuropathy, increased length of the hallux, increased interphalangeal angle, increased body weight, decreased soft tissue thickness and pes planus are all associated with increased pressure at the hallux (Mueller et al., 2003).

Another common deformity seen in diabetic feet is Charcot's neuroarthropathy. Charcot's foot is characterized by neuropathic fractures of the midfoot region resulting in collapse of the arch of the foot. Involvement of the tarsal joints can cause the plantar surface to become convex resulting in the classic "rocker-bottom" foot. This deformity leads to areas of elevated pressure on skin that is not adapted to tolerate pressure and ultimately leads to ulceration (Mueller et al., 1990). Abnormal perfusion of the bones of the midfoot precipitated by autonomic neuropathy may be an etiologic component (O'Loughlin et al., 2010). Both Charcot deformity and hammer toes have been shown to be independent risk factors for diabetic foot ulcers (Boyko et al., 1999).

2.4 Microvascular factors and ulceration

Adequate vascular supply is essential for healing and ischemia often plays a role in ulceration of the diabetic foot. Wound healing requires an adequate supply of oxygen and nutrients be provided to cells involved in the repair process. Peripheral arterial disease

(PAD) is estimated to occur twice as frequently among persons with DM as those without (Dinh et al.). Lower extremity arterial insufficiency in persons with DM can have both macro- and microvascular components. Probability of healing in diabetic foot ulcers has been shown to be strongly related to severity of peripheral vascular disease (Apelqvist et al., 2011). The reported prevalence of PAD in patients with diabetic foot ulcers ranges from 10% to 60% (Armstrong and Lavery, 1998; Oyibo et al., 2001; Moulik et al., 2003). A multi-center trial in Europe reported an overall PAD prevalence of 49% but this varied from 22 to 73% among various centers (Prompers et al., 2007). Peripheral arterial disease typically affects infrapopliteal vessels specifically the profunda femoris in people with DM (Dinh et al.).

Tissue viability ultimately depends on adequate local blood supply to cells via the microcirculation. Alterations in microcirculation have been implicated in formation of diabetic foot ulcers for some time (Dinh and Veves). Dysfunction in the microcirculation of the diabetic foot is not occlusive in nature but secondary to structural and functional changes (Dinh et al.; Chao and Cheing, 2009). The chronic hyperglycemia brought on by DM leads to intracellular accumulation of glucose inducing alterations in multiple metabolic pathways in vascular and neural tissue. Hyperglycemia is a causative factor in impaired vascular permeability and tone as well as auto regulation of blood flow (Chao and Cheing, 2009). Impaired vasodilatory response to plantar pressure causing tissue ischemia is the common final pathway, according to various theories, of the development of diabetic foot ulcers (Boulton et al., 2000). Diabetic patients (with or without peripheral neuropathy) suffer from various forms of microvascular dysfunction, including abnormal vasomotion (Benbow et al., 1995; Stansberry et al., 1996; Bernardi et al., 1997), impaired vasodilatory response to local heating (Malik et al., 1993; Stansberry et al., 1999), decreased blood flow under or after pressure loading (Fromy et al., 2002; Koitka et al., 2004), endothelial nitric oxide dysfunction (Veves et al., 1998), and attenuated response to sympathetic maneuvers (Aso et al., 1997).

Thickening of basement membranes and reduction in capillary size are structural changes that are more prominent in the lower extremities (Dinh et al.). Functionally, vasoreactivity is impaired via reduction in both endothelium-dependent and non-endothelium dependent vasodilation. Both endothelium- and non-endothelium-dependent vasodilation are impaired in the presence of peripheral neuropathy while PAD primarily affects non-endothelium-dependent vasodilation (Dinh et al.; Veves and King, 2001). Occlusive vascular lesions would be more amenable to surgical intervention while the functional ischemia resulting from dysfunctional vasoreactivity would be less responsive to bypass procedures (Veves et al., 1998). Therefore correction of macrocirculatory issues will not necessarily result in healing of a diabetic foot ulcer or prevention of one in the future (Arora et al., 2002).

Microcirculation in persons with DM can also be adversely affected by the neuropathic impairment of the nerve-axon reflex. Stimulation of the C-nociceptive nerve fibers ordinarily leads to release of local vasodilators such as substance P, bradykinin and calcitonin gene-related peptide (CGRP). These neuropeptides act to produce vasodilation via direct action on vascular smooth muscle or indirectly on mast cells through histamine release. This axon mediated response normally accounts for roughly 1/3 of the endothelium-dependent vasodilation in the foot and forearm (Hamdy et al., 2001). This neurogenic vasodilatory response is impaired in the presence of diabetic peripheral neuropathy and the number of sensory neurons for substance P and CGRP reduced (Levy et al.; Caselli et al., 2003).

2.5 Diabetic foot ulcers and lower extremity amputation

DM increases the risk for lower extremity amputation (LEA) from 2% to 16% depending on study design and the population studied (Adler et al., 1999; Lavery et al., 2003; Resnick et al., 2004; Frykberg et al., 2006). Rates of LEA among persons with DM can be as much as 15 to 40 times higher than their non-DM counterparts (Lavery et al., 1996; Resnick et al., 1999). Incidence rates of all LEAs are 4-7 times higher in men and women with DM than in people without DM (Frykberg et al., 2006). A Dutch study found the incidence rate of initial unilateral LEA was 8 times higher in persons with DM than in persons without DM (Johannesson et al., 2009). Lavery et al. found men with DM were 2.35 times more likely to have an LEA than women with DM (Lavery et al., 1999). In a Native American population with DM, risk of LEA was twice as high for men as women (Resnick et al., 2004). Amputation risk varies among ethnic groups being 1.72 to 2.17 times higher in African Americans than non-Hispanic whites and Hispanics (Lavery et al., 1996) and Native Americans, Hispanic Americans and African Americans having a 1.5 to 2.4 fold increased risk of DM-related LEAs than their age-matched Caucasian counterparts (Lavery et al., 1999; Resnick et al., 2004).

The majority of LEAs due to DM were toe amputations followed by BKAs then AKAs and foot amputations with rates of 2.6, 1.6, and 0.8 per 1000 in 2002 (Centers for Disease Control and Prevention, 2005). Several studies in the US and western Europe in recent years have reported decreasing incidence of LEAs in DM populations particularly in response to implementation of improved diabetes foot care (Krishnan et al., 2008; Schofield et al., 2009). In the 5 year longitudinal study by Canavan et al. (2008), the incidence rate of LEA in persons with DM dropped from 310.5 per 100,000 persons to 75.9 per 100,000. A similar dramatic 62% reduction in incidence of major LEAs and a more modest 40.3% decline in total LEAs over 11 years were reported (Krishnan et al., 2008). However, a large retrospective study utilizing a nationwide sample in England found no significant decrease in incidence of DM-related LEAs from 2004 to 2008 (Vamos et al., 2010). The explanation for the differences in findings may lie in the differences in study design as retrospective studies have been reported to underestimate incidence by 4.2% to 90.6% and misclassify 4.5% to 17.4% of amputations (Rayman et al., 2004).

2.6 Risk factors for diabetes-related amputation

Generally speaking, the same factors involved in ulceration of the diabetic foot can have at least contributory roles in LEAs. PAD, infection, chronic hyperglycemia, and history of previous diabetic foot ulcers or amputation are significant risk factors for amputation. Ischemia is a contributory if not the major factor determining the need for a LEA (Schofield et al., 2006). PAD is an independent risk factor for LEA in people with DM (Adler et al., 1999; Moulik et al., 2003; Davis et al., 2006). Adequate blood supply is necessary for healing and resolution of infection as impaired blood interferes with tissue oxygenation and antibiotic delivery to affected regions. PAD is present in 8% of adults with DM at the time of diagnosis and there is a 3.5 fold risk among men with DM and a 8.6 fold risk among women of developing PAD (Melton et al., 1980; Kannel, 1985). In a study by Moulik et al. (2003), 59% of patients who had LEAs over a 5 year follow-up period had PAD and 5 year amputation rates were higher and times to amputation were shorter in this group. While infection may not be an independent risk factor for LEA is often related to inadequate blood flow and interferes with healing (Reiber et al., 1999).

Chronic hyperglycemia and insulin use, which could be considered a marker for glycemic control, have been shown to be independent risk factors for LEA in persons with DM (Adler et al., 1999; Davis et al., 2006; Adler et al., 2010). Elevated HbA1c is associated with risk of LEA such that for every 1% increase in HbA1c there is an associated 26% to 36% increased risk of LEA (Adler et al., 2010). Positive associations have been observed between glycemia and micro- and macrovascular complications and clinical trials have demonstrated the value of improved glycemic control on microvascular complications (DCCT, 1993; UKPDS, 1998). Data on macrovascular complications and glycemic control is less clear with limited clinical trial data to unequivocally demonstrate that intensive glycemic control reduces risk of LEA (Zoungas et al., 2008; Patel et al., 2009; Adler et al., 2010).

Increased risk of LEA associated with hyperglycemia is thought to be mediated by PAD and peripheral sensory neuropathy. Various biochemical changes resulting from hyperglycemia including glycation, protein kinase C activation, sorbitol and hexosamine pathway activation result in arterial disease, sensory neuropathy, autonomic dysfunction and ultimately deregulation of blood flow (Adler et al., 2010). History of diabetic foot ulcers and previous amputation are both independent predictors of LEAs (Adler et al., 1999; Resnick et al., 2004; Davis et al., 2006). Presence of a diabetic foot ulcer is the single biggest risk factor for nontraumatic amputation in persons with DM and increases the risk of amputation 6-fold (Brem et al., 2006; Davis et al., 2006). A diabetic foot ulcer precedes 85% of major LEAs in individuals with DM (Larsson et al., 1997). The presence of a diabetic foot ulcer alone in a person with DM increases the risk of LEA 7 times relative to patients with Charcot arthropathy alone and diabetic foot ulcers together with Charcot arthropathy increases the risk of LEA 12 times versus Charcot arthropathy alone (Sohn et al., 2010).

2.7 Morbidity and mortality following diabetes-related lower extremity amputation

The causal factors leading to the initial amputation remain in place following LEA and continue to place these individuals at elevated risk for re-ulceration. Re-ulceration risk is higher in those with a previous amputation due to increased pressure on a smaller residual weight bearing area, abnormal pressure distribution on the remaining plantar surface and alterations in bony architecture. Thirty-four percent of amputees re-ulcerate in the first year and 70% after 5 years (Apelqvist et al., 1993). Further amputation is twice as likely in persons with DM than in those without with 22% undergoing another amputation a median of 7 months following initial amputation (Schofield et al., 2006). Re-amputation at a higher level on the residual limb is a function of disease progression, failure to heal, and risk factors that develop as a result of the initial amputation such as alteration in the pressure distribution on the residual weight bearing surface. Age and heel lesions have also been shown to be risk factors for re-amputation (Skoutas et al., 2009). Risk of re-amputation is highest within the first 6 months of initial amputation (Izumi et al., 2006; Skoutas et al., 2009). A re-amputation rate of 21.5% within 18 months was reported by Skoutas et al (2009) and 1 year and 3 year rates of 26.7% and 48.3% by Izumi (2006). Forty percent of subjects with DM in a study by Tentolouris et al. had an ipsilateral or contralateral amputation within an average of about 16 months of the first DM-related LEA (Tentolouris et al., 2004).

Mortality risk following LEA is higher for individuals with DM than those without DM. People with DM had a 55% increased risk of death after amputation compared to those without DM (Schofield et al., 2006). One of the first prospective studies on long-term prognosis following LEA amputation reported 1, 3, and 5 year mortality rates of 15%, 38%, and 68%, respectively for both minor and major amputations combined (Larsson et al., 1997). Almost 10 years later, researchers were still reporting people with DM who underwent LEA had a 55% greater risk of dying than those without DM (Schofield et al., 2006).

3. Management of diabetic foot ulceration

The over-arching goal of healthcare professionals engaged in the management of persons with DM is to successfully intervene in the causal pathway leading to diabetic foot ulcers and ultimately amputation. Management of the diabetic foot can be viewed in 4 phases: prevention, accommodation or adaptation, healing and rehabilitation which unfortunately often circles around to become prevention again in an effort to prevent re-ulceration. The scope of this chapter limits discussion primarily to the healing phase of this process.

Clinical trial data suggest better glycemic control mitigates the microvascular complications of the disease including peripheral neuropathy (DCCT, 1993; UKPDS, 1998). Preventing or delaying onset of peripheral neuropathy and its attendant sensory, motor, and autonomic sequelae is paramount to prevention of diabetic foot ulcers. Peripheral polyneuropathy and the tissue changes it induces: loss of protective sensation; inability to perceive trauma; structural changes leading to deformity and areas prone to excessive pressure; impaired sweat gland function producing dry, atrophic skin, all lead to a foot susceptible to injury.

Once peripheral neuropathy is present, focus of care shifts to managing and successfully adapting to the attendant tissue changes. Patient education on foot care becomes even more critical including routine foot inspection, lubrication of dry skin, avoidance of soaking feet, and appropriate callus and nail management. Adaptive footwear must be provided at frequent intervals to accommodate structural changes and relieve pressure.

3.1 Treatment of diabetic foot ulcers

Healing of DFUs is related to how well the underlying etiologies of neuropathy and ischemia and their consequences are addressed. Traditionally, five elements are considered critical to adequate treatment of diabetic foot disease: off-loading or pressure relief, revascularization when appropriate, debridement, management of infection, and wound care. As the magnitude of diabetic foot disease has continued to grow along with our understanding of wound healing in general and the pathophysiology of DM in particular, wound care strategies have progressed as well and there are an ever growing number of advanced wound care products and therapies available. Some of the more widely available include preventive surgery, negative pressure wound therapy (NPWT), hyperbaric oxygen therapy (HBO), and advanced wound care products such as growth factors and living skin equivalents.

3.2 Off-loading

Diabetic foot ulcers on weight or pressure bearing areas in feet lacking protective sensation must be unloaded or relieved of pressure to facilitate healing. A recent review of off-loading techniques for the diabetic foot by Cavenagh and Bus (2011) notes total contact casting

(TCC) remains the gold standard for off-loading although removable walkers have also been shown to provide a similar degree of pressure relief. Peak pressure reduction in the forefoot is reported to be up to 87% with TCC but only 44% to 64% with cast shoes and forefoot offloading shoes (Cavanagh and Bus, 2011). Rocker bottom outsoles, custom insoles, metatarsal pads and arch supports may reduce forefoot peak pressure 16% to 52% compared to controls (Cavanagh and Bus, 2011).

Effectiveness of an off-loading device must be gauged by both its ability to relieve pressure and patients' adherence to the treatment. TCCs are considered to be effective in part because they essentially coerce patient adherence to treatment. Some of the unloading is achieved by restricting ankle motion and redistributing load to the device itself which may explain why devices that extend only to the ankle are less effective in off-loading the foot than those that reach above the ankle (Cavanagh and Bus, 2011). The majority of evidence for off-loading comes from studies examining uncomplicated neuropathic plantar ulcers. TCC has been shown to be more effective in time to healing than removable devices in some randomized clinical trials while a recent RCT showed similar healing rates between a TCC and an ankle high removable walker (Faglia et al., 2010). Off-loading has been used to treat neuroischemic or infected wounds but success rates are much lower than for purely neuropathic ulcers (Nabuurs-Franssen et al., 2005). TCCs are not in wider use because of potential adverse reactions which include diminished activity level, problems sleeping or driving a car and iatrogenic ulcers from poorly applied casts.

Cavanagh and Bus (2011) summarized the recommendations of the International Working Group on the Diabetic Foot for use of off-loading in management of non-complicated foot ulcers in their review: 1) pressure relief should be part of every treatment plan; 2) TCC and non-removable walkers are preferred but clinicians should be aware of potential adverse effects; 3) forefoot off-loading shoes or cast shoes may be used when the above devices are contraindicated or not tolerated; and 4) conventional or standard footwear should not be used as other devices are more effective.

3.3 Revascularization

Peripheral vascular disease is common in persons with DM and is characterized by impairment at both macro- and microvascular levels. Re-establishing arterial supply is the key to healing ischemic and neuroischemic ulcers. Treatment of peripheral arterial disease involves management of risk factors, medical therapy, and endovascular or open surgery. Smoking cessation, weight loss, and adherence to a low fat diet are all areas in which eliciting patient cooperation is critical for successful management. Antiplatelet therapy, anticoagulation, and LDL lowering drugs may also play a role in treatment. However, many diabetic patients will need re-vascularization to achieve healing. Macrovascular disease is morphologically the same in diabetics and non-diabetics differing only in location with the anterior and posterior tibial and peroneal arteries of the calf being most affected in persons with DM. Surgical options are dependent on whether the vascular disease is supra-inguinal (aorto-iliac) or infra-inguinal (femoro-popliteal-crural) or both ((Ruef et al., 2004). Angioplasty, endoarterectomy, grafting, and by-pass are some available surgical interventions. Vascular surgery may be able to aid in revascularization of an area via restoring flow through larger vessels but will not completely restore the microvascular flow disrupted by structural changes in the basement membranes or functional impairment in microcirculation caused by the disease.

3.4 Debridement

Debridement is necessary for removal of devitalized tissue in order to create a healthier wound bed. Removal of nonviable tissue permits better visualization of the wound base, removes a growth medium for bacteria and stimulates release of growth factors. Sharp debridement is the gold standard for diabetic foot ulcers and is the most efficient method for removing large amounts of tissue quickly. Other types of debridement include autolytic, enzymatic, and biologic.

3.5 Management of infection

All open wounds can potentially provide warm, moist environments attractive to microorganisms and thus run the risk of being colonized making infection difficult to diagnose microscopically. The diagnosis of infection is typically based on the presence of purulent drainage or at least 2 clinical signs of inflammation (warmth, erythema, induration, pain, and tenderness) but as these can be mimicked and obscured by the presence of neuropathy or ischemia; it has been proposed that friable tissue, wound undermining and foul odor be used to indicate infection (Pittet et al., 1999; Edmonds and Foster, 2004). Systemic signs of infection such as fever and leukocytosis are not typically seen with diabetic foot ulcers but when present, signal the infection is likely severe (Cavanagh et al., 2005).

As noted earlier, virtually all wounds are colonized so tissue specimens obtained via biopsy, curettage, or aspiration are preferable to wound swabs because results are more specific and sensitive (Lipsky et al., 2004). The most important pathogens implicated in DFU infections are aerobic gram-positive cocci especially *Staph. Aureus* but also β hemolytic streptococci and coagulase-negative staphylococci. Treatment of infection in bone underlying a diabetic foot ulcer presents a particular challenge. Osteomyelitis should be considered present if bone is visible in the wound or palpable with a probe. Bone scans and labeled white blood cell scans are more sensitive for detecting osteomyelitis than plain film x-rays but relatively non-specific and less accurate than MRI. A bone biopsy preferably obtained percutaneously or by surgical debridement is the gold standard test for osteomyelitis but carries the obvious risks associated with invasive testing.

3.6 Wound care

In one sense, care of a wound on a diabetic foot is no different from the care of any other wound in that the basic tenets of wound care apply. A healthy wound environment must be created by removing necrotic tissue, managing bacterial load and maintaining an appropriate moisture balance. Effective use of wound dressings provides a wound environment that encourages angiogenesis, prevents tissue dehydration, promotes cell migration and interaction of growth factors with target cells (Field, 1994). Wound care products are available in a dazzling array to address all aspects of wound bed management but there are unfortunately few RCTs available to support clinical effectiveness. However, it is important to note that local wound care is insufficient for healing of diabetic foot ulcers in most cases unless the underlying diabetic etiologic factors are addressed.

3.7 Preventive surgery

Surgery may be necessary to correct biomechanical faults and/or distribute pressure in order to promote healing of a diabetic foot ulcer or prevent re-ulceration. Prophylactic surgery to correct deformities prior to ulceration has been advocated as a preventive strategy (Mueller et al., 2003). Ulcer healing can be accelerated and recurrence prevented in feet with toe deformities by utilization of extensor tenotomy (Margolis et al., 2005). Achilles tendon lengthening reduces pressure under the metatarsal heads and promotes ulcer healing but the concomitant gait alteration increases the risk of heel ulcers prompting these authors to recommend avoiding this procedure in individuals with complete sensory loss of the heel pad (Holstein et al., 2004). Metatarsal osteotomy and metatarsal head resection have been advocated by some but these procedures pose the risk of secondary ulceration or Charcot foot formation (Petrov et al., 1996; Fleischli et al., 1999). RCTs comparing surgical and non-surgical management of DFUs are scarce. Finally, any surgery is producing a wound that carries a risk of non-healing and infection.

3.8 Negative pressure wound therapy

Negative pressure wound therapy utilizes a vacuum pump to create a subatmospheric wound environment. A wound dressing, typically an open cell foam or saline moistened gauze is placed in the wound cavity to distribute the pressure. A tube connects the cavity to the vacuum pump and the area is sealed with an adhesive film. The portable vacuum pump exerts and maintains a negative pressure in the range of about 50 to 125 mmHg. The mechanical force exerted by the vacuum on the wound surface creates microstrain induced microdeformations of the wound tissue which in turn promotes cellular stretch and proliferation. Micromechanical forces resulting from the negative pressure encourage cell proliferation and migration, extracellular matrix deposition and gene expression. The subatmospheric pressure also prompts angiogenesis and reduction in local edema, excess interstitial fluid, increased lymphatic flow, and removal of waste by-products (Krasner Diane L; Rodeheaver, 2007). Authors of an RCT examining the effectiveness of NPWT in DFUs reported the incidence of secondary amputation was significantly lower when using NPWT (4.1%) compared to moist wound care (10.2%) (Blume et al., 2008). Increased granulation tissue formation and decreased healing times were seen in a RCT of 162 diabetic subjects with partial foot amputations (Armstrong et al., 2005).

3.9 Hyperbaric oxygen therapy

Recognizing that a fundamental problem in non-healing wounds was hypoxia; researchers sought ways to raise tissue oxygen levels. Hyperbaric oxygen therapy entails breathing 100% oxygen pressurized typically between 2.0 and 2.5 absolute atmospheres or ATAs (1 ATA = atmospheric pressure at sea level) with the goal of raising the oxygen partial pressure to about 1500 mmHg. Oxygen delivery to the wound is subsequently improved by the HBO-provided increase in blood oxygen concentration. In addition, HBO has been shown stimulate angiogenesis, enhance neutrophil killing ability, and stimulate fibroblast activity and collagen synthesis (Hunt and Pai, 1972; Knighton et al., 1986). A number of RCTs supporting the efficacy of HBO in the treatment of DFUs have been published but there are still questions about its therapeutic benefits (Tecilazich et al., 2011) and its non-selective use among persons with diabetic foot ulcers (Londahl et al., 2011).

3.10 Advanced wound care products

Wound healing is regulated at least in part by the action of growth factors at various points in the healing cascade. Growth factors are polypeptides transiently produced by cells that exert hormone-like effects on other cells by binding to surface receptors and activating cellular proliferation and differentiation. Some of the more important growth factors for healing include platelet-derived growth factor, transforming growth factor alpha and beta, fibroblast growth factor and epithelial growth factor. Many growth factors are decreased in chronic diabetic foot ulcers. An example of a topically applied growth factor is the genetically engineered, recombinant DNA platelet-derived growth factor, becaplermin. Becaplermin addresses the lack of platelet-derived growth factor-BB and stimulates chemotaxis and mitogenesis of neutrophils, fibroblasts and monocytes. On a cautionary note, the FDA issued a black box warning for this product citing increased risk of death from cancer in patients who used 3 or more tubes of the product.

Living skin equivalents (LSE) comprise another class of advanced local wound care products that is rapidly expanding. These tissue-engineered skins offer notable advantages over skin grafting: because their use is non-invasive, anesthesia is not required, they can be applied in out-patient settings and potential donor site complications such as infection and scarring are avoided. Bioengineered tissue acts not only as a biological dressing but also facilitates healing by filling the wound with extracellular matrix and inducing the expression of growth factors and cytokines which in turn facilitate the healing cascade. LSEs are available for epidermal, dermal and composite (dermal and epidermal) wounds. Autologous grafts or autografts are comprised of cells harvested from the patient then cultured. Grafts from these master cell cultures can then be subcultured into sheets and obtained from an unrelated donor. Allergenic grafts are tissue engineered from neonatal fibroblasts and keratinocytes.

4. Conclusion

The complexity and multifaceted nature of diabetic foot ulceration requires a coordinated approach by a multidisciplinary team of healthcare providers yet even when optimal treatment is provided one study suggests only about 50% of diabetic foot ulcers will be healed after 12-20 weeks. Experts suggest the most cost-effective way to approach wound care in this population is through implementation of a standardized treatment regimen with assessment of wound healing rate every 4 weeks. Advanced wound care therapies should be reserved for those diabetic foot ulcers with healing rates < 50% after 4 weeks. All diabetic foot ulcers are initially managed with a standardized treatment regime and re-assessed every 4 weeks. Wounds healing at a rate of 50% or more continue with the standard regimen while those healing at a rate below 50% receive more aggressive treatment approaches. It should be emphasized that these advanced wound care therapies are in addition to the standard treatments of offloading, debridement, ischemia and infection management.

Diabetic foot ulcers and LEAs present challenges to clinicians not only as serious but ultimately preventable sources of pain, suffering and death to individuals but as virtual black holes to health care resources. A clearer understanding of the nature of these complications and the threats they pose will enable healthcare providers to make informed decisions and implement best practices of care.

5. Acknowledgment

This study was supported by the Oklahoma Center for the Advancement of Science and Technology (OCAST HR09-048).

6. References

Abbott, C. A., A. L. Carrington, H. Ashe, S. Bath, L. C. Every, et al. (2002). "The North-West Diabetes Foot Care Study: incidence of, and risk factors for, new diabetic foot ulceration in a community-based patient cohort." Diabetic Medicine 19(5): 377-384.

Abouaesha, F., C. H. van Schie, G. D. Griffths, R. J. Young and A. J. Boulton (2001). "Plantar tissue thickness is related to peak plantar pressure in the high-risk diabetic foot." Diabetes Care 24(7): 1270-1274.

Adler, A., S. Erqou, T. Lima and A. Robinson (2010). "Association between glycated haemoglobin and the risk of lower extremity amputation in patients with diabetes mellitusâ€"review and meta-analysis." Diabetologia 53(5): 840-849.

Adler, A. I., E. J. Boyko, J. H. Ahroni and D. G. Smith (1999). "Lower-extremity amputation in diabetes. The independent effects of peripheral vascular disease, sensory neuropathy, and foot ulcers." Diabetes Care 22(7): 1029-1035.

Andreassen, C. S., J. Jakobsen and H. Andersen (2006). "Muscle Weakness: A Progressive Late Complication in Diabetic Distal Symmetric Polyneuropathy." Diabetes 55(3): 806-812.

Apelqvist, J., T. Elgzyri, J. Larsson, M. Londahl, P. Nyberg, et al. (2011). "Factors related to outcome of neuroischemic/ischemic foot ulcer in diabetic patients." Journal of Vascular Surgery 53(6): 1582-1588.

Apelqvist, J., J. Larsson and C. D. Agardh (1993). "Long-term prognosis for diabetic patients with foot ulcers." Journal of Internal Medicine 233(6): 485-491.

Armstrong, D. G. and L. A. Lavery (1998). "Elevated peak plantar pressures in patients who have Charcot arthropathy." Journal of Bone & Joint Surgery - American Volume 80(3): 365-369.

Armstrong, D. G., L. A. Lavery and C. Diabetic Foot Study (2005). "Negative pressure wound therapy after partial diabetic foot amputation: a multicentre, randomised controlled trial." Lancet 366(9498): 1704-1710.

Armstrong, D. G., L. A. Lavery and L. B. Harkless (1998). "Validation of a diabetic wound classification system. The contribution of depth, infection, and ischemia to risk of amputation." Diabetes Care 21(5): 855-859.

Arora, S., F. Pomposelli, F. W. LoGerfo and A. Veves (2002). "Cutaneous microcirculation in the neuropathic diabetic foot improves significantly but not completely after successful lower extremity revascularization." Journal of Vascular Surgery 35(3): 501-505.

Aso, Y., T. Inukai and Y. Takemura (1997). "Evaluation of skin vasomotor reflexes in response to deep inspiration in diabetic patients by laser Doppler flowmetry. A new approach to the diagnosis of diabetic peripheral autonomic neuropathy." Diabetes Care 20(8): 1324-1328.

Benbow, S. J., D. W. Pryce, K. Noblett, I. A. MacFarlane, P. S. Friedmann, et al. (1995). "Flow motion in peripheral diabetic neuropathy." Clinical Science 88(2): 191-196.

Bernardi, L., M. Rossi, S. Leuzzi, E. Mevio, G. Fornasari, et al. (1997). "Reduction of 0.1 Hz microcirculatory fluctuations as evidence of sympathetic dysfunction in insulin-dependent diabetes." Cardiovascular Research 34(1): 185-191.

Blume, P. A., J. Walters, W. Payne, J. Ayala and J. Lantis (2008). "Comparison of negative pressure wound therapy using vacuum-assisted closure with advanced moist wound therapy in the treatment of diabetic foot ulcers: a multicenter randomized controlled trial." Diabetes Care 31(4): 631-636.

Boulton, A. J., H. Connor and P. R. Cavanagh (2000). The Foot in Diabetes. New York, NY, John Wiley & Sons, Inc.

Boulton, A. J., R. S. Kirsner and L. Vileikyte (2004). "Clinical practice. Neuropathic diabetic foot ulcers. [Review] [54 refs]." New England Journal of Medicine 351(1): 48-55.

Boulton, A. J. M., L. Vileikyte, G. Ragnarson-Tennvall and J. Apelqvist (2005). "The global burden of diabetic foot disease." Lancet 366(9498): 1719-1724.

Boyko, E. J., J. H. Ahroni, V. Cohen, K. M. Nelson and P. J. Heagerty "Prediction of diabetic foot ulcer occurrence using commonly available clinical information: the Seattle Diabetic Foot Study." Diabetes Care 29(6): 1202-1207.

Boyko, E. J., J. H. Ahroni, V. Stensel, R. C. Forsberg, D. R. Davignon, et al. (1999). "A prospective study of risk factors for diabetic foot ulcer. The Seattle Diabetic Foot Study." Diabetes Care 22(7): 1036-1042.

Brem, H., P. Sheehan, H. J. Rosenberg, J. S. Schneider and A. J. M. Boulton (2006). "Evidence-based protocol for diabetic foot ulcers." Plastic & Reconstructive Surgery 117(7 Suppl): 193S-209S; discussion 210S-211S.

Brownlee, M., A. Cerami and H. Vlassara (1988). "Advanced glycosylation end products in tissue and the biochemical basis of diabetic complications." New England Journal of Medicine 318(20): 1315-1321.

Bus, S. A., M. Maas, A. L. H. De Lange, R. P. J. Michels and M. Levi (2005). "Elevated plantar pressures in neuropathic diabetic patients with claw/hammer toe deformity." Journal of Biomechanics 38(9): 1918-1925.

Bus, S. A., M. Maas, R. P. Michels and M. Levi (2009). "Role of intrinsic muscle atrophy in the etiology of claw toe deformity in diabetic neuropathy may not be as straightforward as widely believed." Diabetes Care 32(6): 1063-1067.

Caselli, A., J. Rich, T. Hanane, L. Uccioli and A. Veves (2003). "Role of C-nociceptive fibers in the nerve axon reflex-related vasodilation in diabetes." Neurology 60(2): 297-300.

Cavanagh, P. R. and S. A. Bus (2011). "Off-loading the diabetic foot for ulcer prevention and healing." Plastic & Reconstructive Surgery 127: Suppl-256S.

Cavanagh, P. R., B. A. Lipsky, A. W. Bradbury and G. Botek (2005). "Treatment for diabetic foot ulcers." Lancet 366(9498): 1725-1735.

Centers for Disease Control and Prevention, A. (2005). "Data and Trends: National Diabetes Surveillance System." National Center for Chronic Disease Prevention and Health Promotion 2006.

Chao, C. Y. L. and G. L. Y. Cheing (2009). "Microvascular dysfunction in diabetic foot disease and ulceration." Diabetes/Metabolism Research and Reviews 25(7): 604-614.

D'Ambrogi, E., C. Giacomozzi, V. Macellari and L. Uccioli (2005). "Abnormal foot function in diabetic patients: the altered onset of Windlass Mechanism." Diabet Med 22(12): 1713-1719.

Davis, W. A., P. E. Norman, D. G. Bruce and T. M. E. Davis (2006). "Predictors, consequences and costs of diabetes-related lower extremity amputation complicating type 2 diabetes: the Fremantle Diabetes Study." Diabetologia 49(11): 2634-2641.

DCCT (1993). "The effect of intensive treatment of diabetes on the development and progression of long-term complications in insulin-dependent diabetes mellitus. The Diabetes Control and Complications Trial Research Group." New England Journal of Medicine 329(14): 977-986.

Delbridge, L., P. Perry, S. Marr, N. Arnold, D. K. Yue, et al. (1988). "Limited joint mobility in the diabetic foot: relationship to neuropathic ulceration." Diabetic Medicine 5(4): 333-337.

Dinh, T., S. Scovell and A. Veves "Peripheral arterial disease and diabetes: a clinical update." International Journal of Lower Extremity Wounds 8(2): 75-81.

Dinh, T. and A. Veves "Microcirculation of the diabetic foot." Current Pharmaceutical Design 11(18): 2301-2309.

Edmonds, M. and A. Foster (2004). "The use of antibiotics in the diabetic foot." American Journal of Surgery 187(5A): 25S-28S.

Faglia, E., C. Caravaggi, G. Clerici, A. Sganzaroli, V. Curci, et al. (2010). "Effectiveness of removable walker cast versus nonremovable fiberglass off-bearing cast in the healing of diabetic plantar foot ulcer: a randomized controlled trial." Diabetes Care 33(7): 1419-1423.

Field, F. K. M. (1994). "Overview of wound healing in a moist environment." American Journal of Surgery 167: 2S-6S.

Fleischli, J. E., R. B. Anderson and W. H. Davis (1999). "Dorsiflexion metatarsal osteotomy for treatment of recalcitrant diabetic neuropathic ulcers." Foot & Ankle International 20(2): 80-85.

Fromy, B., P. Abraham, C. Bouvet, B. Bouhanick, P. Fressinaud, et al. (2002). "Early decrease of skin blood flow in response to locally applied pressure in diabetic subjects." Diabetes 51(4): 1214-1217.

Frykberg, R. G., D. G. Armstrong, J. Giurini, A. Edwards, M. Kravette, et al. (2006). "Diabetic foot disorders: a clinical practice guideline. American College of Foot and Ankle Surgeons." Journal of Foot & Ankle Surgery 39(5 Suppl): S1-60.

Frykberg, R. G., L. A. Lavery, H. Pham, C. Harvey, L. Harkless, et al. (1998). "Role of neuropathy and high foot pressures in diabetic foot ulceration." Diabetes Care 21(10): 1714-1719.

Gershater, M. A., M. Londahl, P. Nyberg, J. Larsson, J. Thorne, et al. (2009). "Complexity of factors related to outcome of neuropathic and neuroischaemic/ischaemic diabetic foot ulcers: a cohort study." Diabetologia 52(3): 398-407.

Ghanassia, E., L. Villon, J. F. Thuan Dit Dieudonne, C. Boegner, A. Avignon, et al. (2008). "Long-term outcome and disability of diabetic patients hospitalized for diabetic foot ulcers: a 6.5-year follow-up study." Diabetes Care 31(7): 1288-1292.

Giacomozzi, C., E. D'Ambrogi, S. Cesinaro, V. Macellari and L. Uccioli "Muscle performance and ankle joint mobility in long-term patients with diabetes." BMC Musculoskeletal Disorders 9: 99.

Global Lower Extremity Amputation Study, G. (2000). "Epidemiology of lower extremity amputation in centres in Europe, North America and East Asia. The Global Lower Extremity Amputation Study Group." British Journal of Surgery 87(3): 328-337.

Greenman, R. L., L. Khaodhiar, C. Lima, T. Dinh, J. M. Giurini, et al. (2005). "Foot Small Muscle Atrophy Is Present Before the Detection of Clinical Neuropathy." Diabetes Care 28(6): 1425-1430.

Hamdy, O., K. Abou-Elenin, F. W. LoGerfo, E. S. Horton and A. Veves (2001). "Contribution of nerve-axon reflex-related vasodilation to the total skin vasodilation in diabetic patients with and without neuropathy." Diabetes Care 24(2): 344-349.

Holewski, J. J., K. M. Moss, R. M. Stess, P. M. Graf and C. Grunfeld (1989). "Prevalence of foot pathology and lower extremity complications in a diabetic outpatient clinic. [Review] [39 refs]." Journal of Rehabilitation Research & Development 26(3): 35-44.

Holstein, P., M. Lohmann, M. Bitsch and B. Jorgensen (2004). "Achilles tendon lengthening, the panacea for plantar forefoot ulceration?" Diabetes/Metabolism Research Reviews 20 Suppl 1: S37-40.

Hunt, T. K. and M. P. Pai (1972). "The effect of varying ambient oxygen tensions on wound metabolism and collagen synthesis." Surgery, Gynecology & Obstetrics 135(4): 561-567.

Izumi, Y., K. Satterfield, S. Lee and L. B. Harkless (2006). "Risk of reamputation in diabetic patients stratified by limb and level of amputation: a 10-year observation." Diabetes Care 29(3): 566-570.

Johannesson, A., G.-U. Larsson, N. Ramstrand, A. Turkiewicz, A.-B. Wirehn, et al. (2009). "Incidence of lower-limb amputation in the diabetic and nondiabetic general population: a 10-year population-based cohort study of initial unilateral and contralateral amputations and reamputations." Diabetes Care 32(2): 275-280.

Kannel, W. B. (1985). "Framingham study insights on diabetes and cardiovascular disease." Clinical Chemistry 57(2): 338-339.

Knighton, D. R., B. Halliday and T. K. Hunt (1986). "Oxygen as an antibiotic. A comparison of the effects of inspired oxygen concentration and antibiotic administration on in vivo bacterial clearance." Archives of Surgery 121(2): 191-195.

Koitka, A., P. Abraham, B. Bouhanick, D. Sigaudo-Roussel, C. Demiot, et al. (2004). "Impaired pressure-induced vasodilation at the foot in young adults with type 1 diabetes." Diabetes 53(3): 721-725.

Krasner Diane L; Rodeheaver, G. T. S., R Gary, Ed. (2007). Chronic Wound Care: A clinical source book for healthcare professionals. Malvern, PA, HMP Communications.

Krishnan, S., F. Nash, N. Baker, D. Fowler and G. Rayman (2008). "Reduction in diabetic amputations over 11 years in a defined U.K. population: benefits of multidisciplinary team work and continuous prospective audit." Diabetes Care 31(1): 99-101.

Landsman, A. S., D. F. Meaney, R. S. Cargill, 2nd, E. J. Macarak and L. E. Thibault (1995). "1995 William J. Stickel Gold Award. High strain rate tissue deformation. A theory on the mechanical etiology of diabetic foot ulcerations." Journal of the American Podiatric Medical Association 85(10): 519-527.

Larsson, J., C. D. Agardh, J. Apelqvist and A. Stenstrom (1997). "Long-term prognosis after healed amputation in patients with diabetes." Clinical Orthopaedics & Related Research(350): 149-158.

Lavery, L. A., D. G. Armstrong, R. P. Wunderlich, J. Tredwell and A. J. M. Boulton (2003). "Diabetic foot syndrome: evaluating the prevalence and incidence of foot pathology in Mexican Americans and non-Hispanic whites from a diabetes disease management cohort." Diabetes Care 26(5): 1435-1438.

Lavery, L. A., H. R. Ashry, W. van Houtum, J. A. Pugh, L. B. Harkless, et al. (1996). "Variation in the incidence and proportion of diabetes-related amputations in minorities." Diabetes Care 19(1): 48-52.

Lavery, L. A., W. H. van Houtum, H. R. Ashry, D. G. Armstrong and J. A. Pugh (1999). "Diabetes-related lower-extremity amputations disproportionately affect Blacks and Mexican Americans." Southern Medical Journal 92(6): 593-599.

Levy, D. M., S. S. Karanth, D. R. Springall and J. M. Polak "Depletion of cutaneous nerves and neuropeptides in diabetes mellitus: an immunocytochemical study." Diabetologia 32(7): 427-433.

Lipsky, B. A., A. R. Berendt, H. G. Deery, J. M. Embil, W. S. Joseph, et al. (2004). "Diagnosis and treatment of diabetic foot infections.[Reprint in Plast Reconstr Surg. 2006 Jun;117(7 Suppl):212S-238S; PMID: 16799390]." Clinical Infectious Diseases 39(7): 885-910.

Londahl, M., K. Fagher and P. Katzman (2011). "What is the role of hyperbaric oxygen in the management of diabetic foot disease?" Current Diabetes Reports 11(4): 285-293.

Malik, R. A., S. Tesfaye, S. D. Thompson, A. Veves, A. K. Sharma, et al. (1993). "Endoneurial localisation of microvascular damage in human diabetic neuropathy." Diabetologia 36(5): 454-459.

Margolis, D. J., L. Allen-Taylor, O. Hoffstad and J. A. Berlin (2005). "Healing diabetic neuropathic foot ulcers: are we getting better?" Diabetic Medicine 22(2): 172-176.

Melton, L. J., 3rd, K. M. Macken, P. J. Palumbo and L. R. Elveback (1980). "Incidence and prevalence of clinical peripheral vascular disease in a population-based cohort of diabetic patients." Diabetes Care 3(6): 650-654.

Morris, A. D., R. McAlpine, D. Steinke, D. I. Boyle, A. R. Ebrahim, et al. (1998). "Diabetes and lower-limb amputations in the community. A retrospective cohort study. DARTS/MEMO Collaboration. Diabetes Audit and Research in Tayside Scotland/Medicines Monitoring Unit." Diabetes Care 21(5): 738-743.

Moulik, P. K., R. Mtonga and G. V. Gill (2003). "Amputation and mortality in new-onset diabetic foot ulcers stratified by etiology." Diabetes Care 26(2): 491-494.

Mueller, M. J., M. Hastings, P. K. Commean, K. E. Smith, T. K. Pilgram, et al. (2003). "Forefoot structural predictors of plantar pressures during walking in people with diabetes and peripheral neuropathy." Journal of Biomechanics 36(7): 1009-1017.

Mueller, M. J., S. D. Minor, J. E. Diamond and V. P. Blair, III (1990). "Relationship of foot deformity to ulcer location in patients with diabetes mellitus." Physical Therapy 70(6): 356-362.

Mueller, M. J., D. R. Sinacore, M. K. Hastings, M. J. Strube and J. E. Johnson (2003). "Effect of Achilles tendon lengthening on neuropathic plantar ulcers. A randomized clinical trial." Journal of Bone & Joint Surgery - American Volume 85-A(8): 1436-1445.

Murray, H. J., M. J. Young, S. Hollis and A. J. Boulton (1996). "The association between callus formation, high pressures and neuropathy in diabetic foot ulceration." Diabetic Medicine 13(11): 979-982.

Nabuurs-Franssen, M. H., R. Sleegers, M. S. P. Huijberts, W. Wijnen, A. P. Sanders, et al. (2005). "Total contact casting of the diabetic foot in daily practice: a prospective follow-up study." Diabetes Care 28(2): 243-247.

Nube, V. L., L. Molyneaux and D. K. Yue (2006). "Biomechanical risk factors associated with neuropathic ulceration of the hallux in people with diabetes mellitus." Journal of the American Podiatric Medical Association 96(3): 189-197.

O'Loughlin, A., C. McIntosh, S. F. Dinneen and T. O'Brien (2010). "Review paper: basic concepts to novel therapies: a review of the diabetic foot. [Review] [118 refs]." International Journal of Lower Extremity Wounds 9(2): 90-102.

Oyibo, S. O., E. B. Jude, I. Tarawneh, H. C. Nguyen, D. G. Armstrong, et al. (2001). "The effects of ulcer size and site, patient's age, sex and type and duration of diabetes on the outcome of diabetic foot ulcers." Diabetic Medicine 18(2): 133-138.

Patel, A., S. MacMahon, J. Chalmers, B. Neal, L. Billot, et al. (2009). "Intensive blood glucose control and vascular outcomes in patients with type 2 diabetes." New England Journal of Medicine 358(24): 2560-2572.

Petrov, O., M. Pfeifer, M. Flood, W. Chagares and C. Daniele (1996). "Recurrent plantar ulceration following pan metatarsal head resection." Journal of Foot & Ankle Surgery 35(6): 573-577; discussion 602.

Pittet, D., B. Wyssa, C. Herter-Clavel, K. Kursteiner, J. Vaucher, et al. (1999). "Outcome of diabetic foot infections treated conservatively: a retrospective cohort study with long-term follow-up." Archives of Internal Medicine 159(8): 851-856.

Prompers, L., M. Huijberts, J. Apelqvist, E. Jude, A. Piaggesi, et al. (2007). "High prevalence of ischaemia, infection and serious comorbidity in patients with diabetic foot disease in Europe. Baseline results from the Eurodiale study." Diabetologia 50(1): 18-25.

Rayman, G., S. T. M. Krishnan, N. R. Baker, A. M. Wareham and A. Rayman (2004). "Are we underestimating diabetes-related lower-extremity amputation rates? Results and benefits of the first prospective study." Diabetes Care 27(8): 1892-1896.

Reiber, G. E., L. Vileikyte, E. J. Boyko, M. del Aguila, D. G. Smith, et al. (1999). "Causal pathways for incident lower-extremity ulcers in patients with diabetes from two settings." Diabetes Care 22(1): 157-162.

Resnick, H. E., E. A. Carter, J. M. Sosenko, S. J. Henly, R. R. Fabsitz, et al. (2004). "Incidence of lower-extremity amputation in American Indians: the Strong Heart Study." Diabetes Care 27(8): 1885-1891.

Resnick, H. E., P. Valsania and C. L. Phillips (1999). "Diabetes mellitus and nontraumatic lower extremity amputation in black and white Americans: the National Health and Nutrition Examination Survey Epidemiologic Follow-up Study, 1971-1992." Archives of Internal Medicine 159(20): 2470-2475.

Ribu, L., B. R. Hanestad, T. Moum, K. Birkeland and T. Rustoen (2007). "A comparison of the health-related quality of life in patients with diabetic foot ulcers, with a diabetes group and a nondiabetes group from the general population." Quality of Life Research 16(2): 179-189.

Ruef, J., M. Hofmann and J. Haase (2004). "Endovascular interventions in iliac and infrainguinal occlusive artery disease." Journal of Interventional Cardiology 17(6): 427-435.

Salsich, G. B., M. J. Mueller, M. K. Hastings, D. R. Sinacore, M. J. Strube, et al. (2005). "Effect of Achilles tendon lengthening on ankle muscle performance in people with diabetes mellitus and a neuropathic plantar ulcer." Physical Therapy 85(1): 34-43.

Schofield, C. J., G. Libby, G. M. Brennan, R. R. MacAlpine, A. D. Morris, et al. (2006). "Mortality and hospitalization in patients after amputation: a comparison between patients with and without diabetes." Diabetes Care 29(10): 2252-2256.

Schofield, C. J., N. Yu, A. S. Jain and G. P. Leese (2009). "Decreasing amputation rates in patients with diabetes-a population-based study." Diabetic Medicine 26(8): 773-777.

Singh, N., D. G. Armstrong and B. A. Lipsky (2005). "Preventing foot ulcers in patients with diabetes." JAMA 293(2): 217-228.

Skoutas, D., N. Papanas, G. S. Georgiadis, V. Zervas, C. Manes, et al. (2009). "Risk factors for ipsilateral reamputation in patients with diabetic foot lesions." International Journal of Lower Extremity Wounds 8(2): 69-74.

Smith, D. G., B. C. Barnes, A. K. Sands, E. J. Boyko and J. H. Ahroni (1997). "Prevalence of radiographic foot abnormalities in patients with diabetes." Foot & Ankle International 18(6): 342-346.

Sohn, M.-W., R. M. Stuck, M. Pinzur, T. A. Lee and E. Budiman-Mak (2010). "Lower-extremity amputation risk after charcot arthropathy and diabetic foot ulcer." Diabetes Care 33(1): 98-100.

Stansberry, K. B., H. R. Peppard, L. M. Babyak, G. Popp, P. M. McNitt, et al. (1999). "Primary nociceptive afferents mediate the blood flow dysfunction in non-glabrous (hairy) skin of type 2 diabetes: a new model for the pathogenesis of microvascular dysfunction." Diabetes Care 22(9): 1549-1554.

Stansberry, K. B., S. A. Shapiro, M. A. Hill, P. M. McNitt, M. D. Meyer, et al. (1996). "Impaired peripheral vasomotion in diabetes." Diabetes Care 19(7): 715-721.

Sun, P. C., H. D. Lin, S. H. Jao, R. C. Chan, M. J. Kao, et al. (2008). "Thermoregulatory sudomotor dysfunction and diabetic neuropathy develop in parallel in at-risk feet." Diabetic Medicine 25(4): 413-418.

Tecilazich, F., T. Dinh and A. Veves (2011). "Treating diabetic ulcers. [Review]." Expert Opinion on Pharmacotherapy 12(4): 593-606.

Tentolouris, N., S. Al-Sabbagh, M. G. Walker, A. J. M. Boulton and E. B. Jude (2004). "Mortality in diabetic and nondiabetic patients after amputations performed from 1990 to 1995: a 5-year follow-up study." Diabetes Care 27(7): 1598-1604.

Tentolouris, N., K. Marinou, P. Kokotis, A. Karanti, E. Diakoumopoulou, et al. (2009). "Sudomotor dysfunction is associated with foot ulceration in diabetes." Diabetic Medicine 26(3): 302-305.

Tesfaye, S., A. J. M. Boulton, P. J. Dyck, R. Freeman, M. Horowitz, et al. (2010). "Diabetic Neuropathies: Update on Definitions, Diagnostic Criteria, Estimation of Severity, and Treatments." Diabetes Care 33(10): 2285-2293.

UKPDS (1998). "Intensive blood-glucose control with sulphonylureas or insulin compared with conventional treatment and risk of complications in patients with type 2 diabetes (UKPDS 33). UK Prospective Diabetes Study (UKPDS) Group.[Erratum appears in Lancet 1999 Aug 14;354(9178):602]." Lancet 352(9131): 837-853.

Vamos, E. P., A. Bottle, M. E. Edmonds, J. Valabhji, A. Majeed, et al. (2010). "Changes in the incidence of lower extremity amputations in individuals with and without diabetes in England between 2004 and 2008." Diabetes Care 33(12): 2592-2597.

van Schie, C. H. B., A.J. M. Boulton (2006). Biomechanics of the Diabetic Foot: *The Road to Foot Ulceration*. The Diabetic Foot. A. G. Veves, J.M.; LoGerfo, F.W. Totowa, NJ, Humana Press Inc.: 185-200.

Veves, A., C. M. Akbari, J. Primavera, V. M. Donaghue, D. Zacharoulis, et al. (1998). "Endothelial dysfunction and the expression of endothelial nitric oxide synthetase in diabetic neuropathy, vascular disease, and foot ulceration." Diabetes 47(3): 457-463.

Veves, A. and G. L. King (2001). "Can VEGF reverse diabetic neuropathy in human subjects?" Journal of Clinical Investigation 107(10): 1215-1218.

Veves, A., H. J. Murray, M. J. Young and A. J. Boulton (1992). "The risk of foot ulceration in diabetic patients with high foot pressure: a prospective study." Diabetologia 35(7): 660-663.

Vinik, A. I., R. E. Maser, B. D. Mitchell and R. Freeman (2003). "Diabetic autonomic neuropathy. [Review] [192 refs]." Diabetes Care 26(5): 1553-1579.

Wild, S., G. Roglic, A. Green, R. Sicree and H. King (2004). "Global prevalence of diabetes: estimates for the year 2000 and projections for 2030." Diabetes Care 27(5): 1047-1053.

Young, M. J., P. R. Cavanagh, G. Thomas, M. M. Johnson, H. Murray, et al. (1992). "The effect of callus removal on dynamic plantar foot pressures in diabetic patients." Diabetic Medicine 9(1): 55-57.

Zimny, S., H. Schatz and M. Pfohl (2004). "The Role of Limited Joint Mobility in Diabetic Patients With an At-Risk Foot." Diabetes Care 27(4): 942-946.

Zoungas, S., B. E. de Galan, T. Ninomiya, D. Grobbee, P. Hamet, et al. (2008). "Combined effects of routine blood pressure lowering and intensive glucose control on macrovascular and microvascular outcomes in patients with type 2 diabetes: New results from the ADVANCE trial." Diabetes Care 32(11): 2068-2074.

2

Stroke Rehabilitation

Chong Tae Kim
Division of Pediatric Rehabilitation Medicine, The Children's Hospital of Philadelphia, Department of Physical Medicine & Rehabilitation, The University of Pennsylvania, USA

1. Introduction

Stroke is defined a sudden neurological impairment resulting from interruption of the blood supply and brain tissue damage. The most common symptom of a stroke is sudden weakness and/or numbness of the face, arms or legs, most often on one side of the body. Other symptoms include: confusion, difficulty speaking or understanding speech; difficulty seeing with one or both eyes; difficulty walking, dizziness, loss of balance or coordination; severe headache with no known causes; fainting or unconsciousness. Generally stroke means compromise of arterial blood supply (arterial stroke). Venous stroke is very rare in adult but not uncommon in children.

Strokes can be classified as either hemorrhagic or non-hemorrhagic (infarction). This classification helps to decide early therapeutic intervention. Hemorrhagic stroke is not indicated for t-PA (tissue plasminogen activator) protocol. Hemorrhagic stroke is most commonly related with hypertension or aneurysm in adults and with congenital vascular abnormality in children. Non-hemorrhagic stroke is more common than hemorrhagic stroke (8:2) in the United States and European countries[1,2], however a more recent study shows 6:4 ratio[3]. This ratio varies in different races and cultures[4].

The diagnostic procedures of stroke are identical in both adult and children. A meticulous history and neurological examination are the mainstays of diagnosis. Head CT (computerized tomography) is useful to differentiate hemorrhagic and non-hemorrhagic stroke in very acute phase. A brain MRI (magnetic resonance image) is requested if head CT is not diagnostic. Intracranial as well as extracranial vessels can be evaluated by a MRA (magnetic resonance arteriography). MRV (magnetic resonance venography) is indicated for venous stroke diagnosis.

In very acute phase of stroke (within 3 hours), a thrombolytic agent (t-PA) is recommended as a standard treatment for non-hemorrhagic strokes in adult. It decreases mortality and improves functional outcome, in spite of hemorrhagic complications[5].

2. Right versus left hemisphere stroke

Right hemisphere function is to control not only the movement of the left side of the body, but also analyze spatial orientation (distance, depth, position, size, and stereotaxis) and perceptual abilities. Stroke patients with right hemisphere lesion often demonstrate lack of safety awareness and impulsive behaviors. With these complex impairments, they have difficulties in re-learning ADL (activities of daily living). For example, they are unable to read or copy letters, forget to clean their left side body, or ignore to wear assistive devices for activity. Even though they can maintain speech-language function better than patients with left hemisphere stroke patients, they may make errors in grammar.

Major functions of the left hemisphere are to control the movements of the right side of the body and to maintain speech-language function. Patients with left hemispheric strokes sustain right hemiplegia and aphasia. They behave cautiously and need more time to complete the same task compared with right hemispheric stroke patients. Different types of aphasia can occur depending on the specific site of the lesion in the left hemisphere.

It is controversial whether rehabilitation outcomes differ depending on which hemisphere the lesion is occurs[6-8]. Possible reasons for the controversy are different outcome scales, measurement domain, presence of hemi-neglect, and evaluation timing. For example, if the outcome compared is vocational rehabilitation, patients with right hemisphere lesion show better outcome[9]. The higher percentage of patients returning to work with a right hemispheric lesion largely can be explained by preserved speech-language function. However patients with right hemispheric lesions more frequently develop social defects than those with left hemispheric lesions[10]. In contrast, if regaining arm function is measured as a rehabilitation outcome, poorer outcome is reported in right hemispheric lesions[11].

Hemi-neglect develops more commonly in stroke patients who have right hemispheric lesion compared to the left. There is a wide range of incidence reported, because of different evaluation tools and evaluation timing[12,13]. Among patients with right hemispheric lesions, patients with hemi-neglect are more disabled and stay longer at rehabilitation facilities than those without hemi-neglect[14]. Again, one possible reason of controversy in outcomes of patients with stroke between right and left hemispheric lesions is that patients with a concurrent right hemispheric lesion with hemi-neglect has more disability than would be with a right hemispheric lesion alone[15]. Future studies excluding hemi-neglect patients may help clarify the difference in disability between right and left hemiplegia patients[16].

3. Hemorrhagic versus non-hemorrhagic stroke

Stroke prognosis between hemorrhagic and non-hemorrhagic stroke, is another area of controversy[17-19]. It is largely attributed to the timing of outcome measurement and scopes of outcome. Not only matched comparison studies[20,21], but also large population retrospective ones[22-24] consistently showed better and faster functional recovery in hemorrhagic versus non-hemorrhagic stroke at short term outcomes. For long-term outcomes (one year post-stroke), one study reported that there was no difference between hemorrhagic and non-hemorrhagic stroke[22], but another study observed better outcome in non-hemorrhagic stroke[23]. For further study, it is to be considered that 20-40% of initial ischemic infarction may develop hemorrhagic transformation within one week after initial stroke onset. Hemorrhagic transformation may blur the distinction between hemorrhagic and non-hemorrhagic strokes and therefore, the classification based on initial imaging studies can be a source of significant bias.

In summary, hemorrhagic stroke has higher mortality rate than non-hemorrhagic in acute phase and often requires emergent surgical intervention for survival. However, hemorrhagic stroke survivors without significant surgical complications make better functional improvement in early phase of rehabilitation than those with non-hemorrhagic stroke.

4. Impairments and disabilities sequelae to stroke

Severity and types of impairments resulted from a stroke depend on stroke site and lesion size. Most common impairments are 1) motor dysfunction (paralysis of extremity, face, and oropharyngeal muscles), 2) sensory dysfunction (decreased sensation, perception disorder, abnormal sensation), 3) sphincter dysfunction (bowel and bladder incontinence), 4) cognitive dysfunction (anomia, aphasia, dementia), 5) emotional disturbance (depression, apathy).

1. Paralysis of one side of body (hemiplegia): It develops in very early phase of stroke. If stroke lesion is in the right hemisphere, paralysis develops in the left face and the extremity. But stroke lesion located in the right brainstem, develops paralysis in the right face and left extremity. Most patients with stroke complain of flaccid extremity as an initial symptom. The flaccid extremity usually evolves to spastic extremity as part of its natural course. Details of motor function recovery will be described in the follow section (Motor function recovery).
   One side of bulbar muscle paralysis results in oropharyngeal dysfunction (dysphagia). Stroke patient with dysphagia needs non-oral feeding until safe swallowing recovered. Depending on the severity of dysphagia, stroke patient needs nasogastric or gastrostomy/jejunostomy tube feeding. VFSS (videofluorographic swallowing study), also called videofluorographic modified barium swallowing study, is a standard diagnostic test to evaluate swallowing function. Penetration is defined when a bolus moves aberrantly down to the vestibule above the true vocal fold. This may trigger a coughing or a choking reflex after swallowing the bolus. Aspiration occurs when a bolus passes farther down through the true vocal folds and enter into the trachea and lungs. Most of patients with dysphagia return to a regular diet in early post-stroke phase[25, 26]. Compared to other lesions, dysphagia develops more common and less favorable outcome in brainstem stroke, however 88% returned to regular oral intake 4 months after stroke[27]. Tracheostomy increases the risk of aspiration because of the limitation of laryngeal elevation during swallowing. Selection of adequate texture of meals and meticulous monitoring of swallowing are critical to prevent aspiration.
2. Sensory impairment: stroke patients have sensory impairment of peripheral and/or central sensation. Peripheral sensory impairments include hypesthesia/paresthesia, loss of proprioception and position, or loss of pain/temperature. Agraphesthesia and astreognosis is seen in central sensory impairment. Those impairments cause stroke patients to needs more assistance for learning motor and cognitive skills. Reception is the processing of registration of sensations or stimuli which are collected through sensory organs (nose, eye, ear, skin, tongue, joint, or internal organs). Received sensations or stimuli are conveyed to the corresponding primary sensory cortexes. For example, visual sensation reaches occipital cortex via optic pathways. Perception is the next process to interpret the received sensations or stimuli. Perception is higher cortical function than reception and many parts of brain are involved. Details of perception disorder will be discussed in the following perception disorder.

3. Sphincter dysfunction: Double incontinence (both urinary and fecal incontinence) is more common than isolated urinary or fecal incontinence in stroke patients[28]. Even though this impairment resolved during early post-stroke period, persistent urinary incontinence was reported 10-20% at the time of discharge from rehabilitation[28, 29]. The most common type of bladder dysfunction is uninhibited type. It is usually resolved with timed voiding training. Sometimes anti-cholinergic agents (oxybutynin, tolterodine) are indicated to relax bladder. Most of sphincter dysfunction is restored as other functional recovery occurs. Nocturnal incontinence may persist in chronic phase. Unawareness of bladder is a strong negative prognostic factor for urinary incontinence, in addition to cognitive impairment and lower limb dysfunction. It may be a lifelong disability in those with significantly cognitive impaired.
4. Cognitive dysfunction is the most powerful negative factor for outcome. This is most commonly and severely impaired in patients with left hemisphere lesion with aphasia. It is also very closely negatively correlated with returning to work. 38% of stroke patients were found to have cognitive impairment assessed by Mini-Mental State Examination at 3 month post-stroke and more common in elderly (>75 years), low socioeconomic status, and left hemisphere lesion[30]. It has strong correlations with long-term outcome. 30-50% of stroke survivors were categorized in lower levels on most measures of neuropsychological testing and information processing is the most common and the worst deficit[31]. Cognitive impairment and dementia after a stroke can be reduced by adequate treatment of hypertension and acetylcholinesterase inhibitors (donepezil, galantamine, rivastigmine), prescribed to alzheimer's disease, and may be beneficial for cognitive rehabilitation[32, 33]. A randomized placebo-controlled double blind study reports that greater improvement of language function in verbal fluency and repetition was found in patients receiving levedopa than placebo[34]. One open label case study shows rapid improvement in cognitive as well as physical function in three chronic stroke patients with perispinal etanercept[35].
5. Emotional disturbance: Right hemispheric stroke patients sustain behavioral changes, which in turn caused family conflicts with this altered behaviors[36]. A 5 year longitudinal study shows about 30% of stroke survivors sustained depression and 48% were not depressed at any time of evaluation[31, 37]. Also depression was not static, but resolved and newly developed at any time in the 5 year follow-up[37]. High risk factors of depression include stroke severity, unemployment, and cognitive impairment. A patient with depression prior to stroke has 9 times higher risk of post-stroke depression[38]. The frequency of post-stroke apathy is reported 20-25% and commonly conjunct with cognitive impairment and depression[39]. Dopaminergics or neurostimulants (methylphenidate, dexamphetamine) is reportedly beneficial to apathy[40-43].

   Post-stroke depression is a strong negative factor for functional recovery, however there is no standard pharmacological treatment. A double-blind controlled study with fluoxetine and nefiracetam did not support therapeutic effectiveness for either agent[44, 45], however, a matched comparison study with milnacipran revealed effectiveness[46]. The controversy is in part ascribed to uncovered pharmacodynamics of anti-depressant in stroke. Systemic review of pharmacological management of post-stroke depression concludes there is insufficient evidence to support anti-depressant administration for prevention or to improve recovery, but the medications may improve mood in post-stroke depression[47].

5. Perception disorder

Perception is the conscious mental process through the senses of existence and external sensory stimulus. Visual perception disorders are manifested as agnosia, alexia, apraxia, hemi-neglect, spatial disorientation. Hemispatial neglect is synonymous with hemiagnosia, hemi-neglect, unilateral neglect, unilateral inattention. Homonymous hemianopsia differs from visual hemi-neglect. While the former is resulted from the lesion of the visual track and the patient with this impairment uses compensate strategy (for example, head turning), the latter is spatial inattention to one side of body resulted from parietal cortex and one with this impairment does not compensate. Perception disorders impede not only functional recovery, but safety awareness. For example, perceptual disorder of position leads the patient stands with asymmetric weight bearing and affects gross motor function recovery. Patients with right hemisphere stroke predominantly sustain spatial perception disorders. Perceptual training with mirror therapy, prism adaption, eye patch, reportedly improves functional outcomes after stroke, but one large review article showed insufficient supportive data of perceptual intervention (visual field deficits, neglect/inattention, and apraxia were excluded in this study) [48, 49].

Apraxia is the inability to carry out familiar, purposeful tasks without sensory or motor impairment, especially difficult is proper use of an object. Patients with speech apraxia demonstrate incomplete speech with repetition, omission, or distorted words. They are doing well with short simple conversations (How are you? Are you OK?...), but the impairment is exaggerated with long complex sentences. Patients with ideational apraxia have difficulties in coordination of sequential performance. For example, he/she knows how to hold a letter, to put it into an envelope, and to attach a stamp. But when he/she is requested to do these three steps sequentially, he/she cannot do this in the proper order. Clinically, it is manifested as difficulties in eating, dressing, and bathing. A patient with ideomotor apraxia is unable to respond properly to a request or command. He/she knows the name of an object, but not able to use properly. For example, when he/she is asked to brush hair with a comb, the patient demonstrates improper usage of the comb. Constructional apraxia is the inability to copy, draw, or construct simple figures. The patient with this impairment draws a face unproportionally. Dressing apraxia, difficulty in wearing cloths, is a misnomer (not true apraxia). This is resulted from the impairment of spatial perception, which makes it difficult to recognize and match the parts of the body and the cloth correctly.

Pain perception disorder: Central post-stroke pain syndrome (CPSP) is one of devastating complications and formerly called thalamic pain syndrome. It is understood that damaged spinothalamic track may play a key role in pathogenesis, but not always. It may develop independently or jointly with complex regional pain syndrome (CRPS). Clinical findings are very similar to CRPS, however, CPSP is confined to hemiplegic face or limbs only. Both the presence of sensory disturbances and neurpathic pain differentiates CPSP from CRPS. It usually develops 1-3 months after stroke onset, but sometimes develops in a chronic phase. Plain radiographic study is recommended to rule out musculoskeletal lesion of the shoulder or hand. In order to rule out deep vein thrombosis, Doppler ultrasound study is useful. Triple phase bone scan is to be considered if CRPS suspected. Therapeutic options are similar to CRPS. Magnetic motor cortex stimulation[50], vestibular stimulation[51,52], or deep vein stimulations[53] are being tried in some cases.

6. Motor function recovery

Hemiplegia is the most paramount clinical feature, which is described as sided weakness of extremity, facial droop, and slurred speech. Motor function recovery follows stereotypic patterns. It initially develops flaccid hemiplegia during the acute phase. Depending on individual cases, however, flaccid hemiplegia evolves into spastic hemiplegia. It continues to evolve into spastic synergy. Typically, flexion synergy develops in hemiplegic upper extremity and extension synergy in the lower extremity. As the synergy fades, individual movement of joints emerges. The longer the length of time in flaccid hemiplegia, the poorer the prognosis of motor recovery. Motor recovery may stagnate at any phase and may skip phases. Another pattern is that proximal segment of extremity function recovers earlier than distal one. Many patients with stroke sustain typical stereotyped poor dexterity and hemiplegic gait because of residual distal extremity dysfunction. In order to facilitate motor recovery, comprehensive rehabilitation modalities, such as anti-spastic medications, orthotics, and therapeutic exercise are cooperated. Significant motor recovery usually occurs in the first three months after stroke. Further recovery may continue in the next three months but less extensive.

Brunnstrom stage describes the evolution of hemiplegia[54]. Flaccid paralyzed extremity is seen at stage 1; Mild spasticity is appreciated in the flaccid paralyzed extremity at stage 2; The spasticity increases and some self-activated synergic movement of the paralyzed extremity begins at stage 3; Dominant stereotyped self-activated synergic movement of the paralyzed extremity is more prominent at stage 4; decreasing synergic movement pattern with emerging individual movement of the paralyzed extremity is the hall mark of the stage 5; normal movement pattern is seen at stage 6. Not all paralyzed extremity evolves from stage 1 to 6. Depending on stroke severity and recovery potential, the stages may progress quickly or may be skipped. Generally speaking, hemiplegia with short or absent stage 1 has better recovery; the longer the stage 1, the worse prognosis; the lower stage, the poorer outcome, [11, 55-58].

In addition to Brunnstrom stage, motor function recovery tends to begin in the proximal segment and then to progress to the distal segments of the extremity. This tendency is common in both upper and lower extremity. Most of stroke patients are able to move their proximal segments of arms and legs at the time of discharge from inpatient rehabilitation. However, many stroke patients sustain significant paralysis of the distal segments of arm and leg. Because of this residual impairment, most stroke survivors have difficulties to be independent with ADLs and ambulation. Another common finding is that motor recovery of the lower extremity is better than that of the upper extremity. Why is motor recovery of the proximal segments and the lower extremity better than that of the distal segments and the lower extremity? It can be partially explained by topographic distribution in the brain (the cortex corresponding to hand is much larger than one to foot in the brain) and higher developmental hierarchy (hand function develops later than foot function). Compared to the proximal segments or foot function, more neurons and synapses are to be involved to maintain functions of the distal segments or hand.

7. Rehabilitation

The priorities at the acute care unit are both diagnostic as well as therapeutic interventions. Depending on medical conditions (hemorrhagic or non-hemorrhagic lesion, size and site of stroke, underlying health status,...), treatment options are determined. It is suggested that early rehabilitation intervention is necessary, even if diagnostic or therapeutic plan are not completed. At this phase, rehabilitation starts with less intensive approach. Passive range of motion, position changes, stimulation control, safe feeding, and joint contracture prevention are important to prevent impending complications.

Functional improvement is not always parallel with neurological recovery in patients with stroke. Analysis of the Uniform Data System for Medical Rehabilitation (UDSMR) for stroke patients in US from 2000 to 2007 shows decreased a mean length of rehabilitation unit stay from 19.6 days to 16.5 days, decrease a mean FIM (functional independence measurement) at rehabilitation unit from 62.5 to 55.1 (means more functionally dependent patients were admitted to rehabilitation unit), decrease a mean FIM at discharge from rehabilitation unit from 86.4 to 79.8 (means less functionally independent patients were discharged from rehabilitation unit), but the FIM change during rehabilitation stay remained relatively stable[59]. These results reflect that patients with stroke in US admit and discharge earlier than before. Patients with stroke may benefit from early discharge, but by the other hand, early discharge from rehabilitation unit increased the mortality[60].

From an ADL (activities of daily living) standpoint, stair walking (downward more difficult than upward) is the hardest to be improved, and then tub/shower transfer, ambulation, and lower body dressing follow. In contrast, eating is the easiest to be improved, and then grooming, and sphincter control follow.

Poor sitting balance, poor trunk control, urinary incontinence, severity of disability, and old age (>74 years) are poor predictors for independent walking[61]. Standing balance ability is more important than lower extremity strength to achieve better ambulation[62].

In cognitive rehabilitation, problem solving is the most severely impaired and the least potential for recovery after stroke. Learning and memory impairments are most common[10]. Comprehension and expression are less impaired and better improved than memory. Patients with right hemiplegia are more impaired and less likely to improve in cognitive functions than those with left hemiplegia.

Cognitive and speech-language impairment prevents patients with stroke from participation in social activities. Patients with higher cognitive level recover much better than ones with lower level. A study of return to work reports 1) no significant racial differences in left hemisphere infarction, but whites were more likely to return to work in right hemisphere infarction, 2) no significant difference of returning to work between whites and non-whites with left hemisphere infarction, 3) whites with right hemisphere infarction are most likely to return to work, while non-whites with right hemisphere infarction are least likely, 4) patients employed premorbidly at professional or managerial position, younger age group, less severe disability, white race, right hemisphere lesion were more likely to return to work following a cerebral infarction[9].

8. Traditional and new therapeutic approaches to stroke rehabilitation

Traditional physical therapy and occupation therapy are still largely mainstays of the rehabilitation. Many therapeutic techniques to facilitate movement of paralyzed side, based on motor developmental hierarchy, repetition of motor pattern, and task-oriented training.

Abnormal muscle tone leads to abnormal positioning and abnormal movement pattern, and vice versa. To break this vicious cycle, comprehensive rehabilitation should include muscle tone management, proper bracing and positioning, and stimulation control. Repetitive task training is a commonly used in current rehabilitation therapy, but a literature review reported it is not effective in upper extremity motor function[63].

Constraint-induced movement therapy (CIMT or CIT) was introduced with a hypothesis of forceful usage of paralytic arm facilitate neuroplasticity of the brain, which in turn leads to recovery of the arm motor function[64]. There are many supportive reports to its effectiveness[65, 66], however, there is a lack of large randomized controlled study[67]. CIMT is indicated for subjects who have no significant spasticity and some strength of the paralyzed upper extremity. It is not effective in acute phase of stroke[68].

Development in neruoscience and computer technology provides novel ideas to overcome the limitation of traditional rehabilitation for stroke. Originally, robotic treatment was introduced to alleviate the labor-intensive aspects of physical therapy by preinstalled programs to perform a goal-directed movement autonoumously or semi-autonomously[69]. It induces movement of paralyzed limbs by activation of the motor cortex of the side of the lesion and the movement of the limb also activates the motor cortex in a positive feedback. Most of devices are designed to lead task-oriented movement by intensive repetitive patterns. Functional brain MRI studies of robotic treatments, demonstrated an increased activation of the sensorimotor cortex during grasping tasks greater than non-practiced tasks[70]. However, the effectiveness of robotic treatment is still in question[71-73]. It is likely effective for shoulder and elbow function recovery, but may lack effectiveness of hand function improvement.

EEG/MEG-based motor imagery brain-computer interface utilizes neuronal activities of the motor cortex of lesion side while performing motor imagery[74, 75]. Currently combined brain-computer interface with robotic feedback technique is being tried[76].

Virtual reality training, although needs further study, appears to be effective in improvement of motor function[77, 78].

9. Prognostic factors

Generally, poor prognostic factors include prolonged flaccidity of paralyzed limb, right hemisphere lesion with hemi-neglect, cognitive impairment, old age (>74 years), anterior circulation, and large lesion size. Also spouse at home, hypothermia at acute phase, and absent co-morbidities are good predictors[79, 80].

10. Focus on pediatric stroke

Pediatric stroke is classified into infant and childhood stroke. Infant (neonatal or perinatal) stroke is defined as occurring between 28 weeks gestation and 28 days of postnatal age. The incidence is estimated as one in every four thousand live birth per year in the United Sates[81]. Ischemic stroke is twice as common as hemorrhagic stroke. According to a retrospective review, the most common discharge diagnoses conjunction with neonatal stroke included infection, cardiac disorders, and blood disorders. Less than 5% was associated with birth asphyxia[81].

Childhood stroke is defined as occurring between 30 days of postnatal age and 18 years old. The incidence is reported 2-3/100,000 per year in US[81], 2.7/100,000 in Canada (ischemic stroke only)[82], and 13/100,000 in France[83]. Its mortality rate is reported 7-28% and higher in males than females and in blacks than white, respectively. Stroke is less common in children than in adults, but is one of the top ten causes of death in children in the US. It results in one of the leading causes of disability in young generations. The pathophysiology of childhood stroke is same as adults, but underlying premorbidities or etiologies are different. Most of adult stroke patients have pre-existing medical conditions, such as hypertension, diabetes mellitus, hyperlipidemia, arteriosclerosis, heart disease, or obesity, but in contrast one third of child stroke patients do not have any evident pre-existing medical conditions. In childhood stroke, congenital heart disease is the most common known etiology (about 30%), and sickle cell disease is the leading cause of stroke in African American ethnic group. Arteriovenous malformation is the leading cause of hemorrhagic stroke in childhood. Various coagulation disorders-factor V Leiden and prothrombin mutation, protein C and S deficiency, anti-phospholipid antibody, and inherited coagulation abnormalities and arterial vasculitis are related to pediatric strokes. Venous stroke is not uncommon in children. Venous:arterial stroke ratio is 1:4-6 in non-hemorrhagic stroke[84]. Venous stroke develops, when cerebral venous drainage to the internal jugular veins is significantly obstructed by thrombosis in the cerebral venous sinus (sinus venous thrombosis). The obstructed venous drainage consequently impedes arterial supply to the brain. Progressive insufficient arterial supply to the brain eventually leads to ischemia. Because of this slow process, compared with arterial stroke, clinical symptoms and signs progress slowly in venous stroke. High risks of sinus venous thrombosis are head and neck infection (meningitis, mastoiditis), dehydration, coagulation disorder, and perinatal complications. The outcome of a venous stroke is excellent.

The ratio of hemorrhagic to nonhemorrhagic stroke in childhood stroke is about 5:3 in the US[85] . It is understood that the incidence of homorrhagic stroke is higher than adult, but it is similar to a recent stroke registry data[3]. Diagnostic interventions of pediatric stroke are similar to those of adult stroke. In addition, hematologic and metabolic work up for coagulopathy is important. It is not easy to recognize neonatal stroke because of limited clinical presentations. It is partially plausible to explain that patients with hemiplegic cerebral palsy might have unrecognized neonatal stroke. It is supported by the fact that patients with hemiplegic cerebral palsy showed elevated antiphospholipid and/or factor V Leiden mutation than normal control[86-87]. Patients with sickle cell disease has 200-400 times high risk and 50% of recurrence risk by three years.

In order to prevent stroke recurrence, aspirin is recommended for high risk of stroke patients in both adult and children. Apirin used for stroke prophylaxis does not complicate Reye's syndrome in children. Regular brain MRA is suggested to patient with hemorrhagic stroke secondary to aneurysm.

Since human cerebral hemispheres are already specialized at an early stage of development, pediatric stroke patients also demonstrate adult pattern of side specificity for brain lesions[88-89]. Therefore clinical features are side specific and similar to adult stroke.

Outcomes vary among studies because of differences in population characteristics, stroke type, duration of follow-up, and outcomes measurement tools. Long-term outcome study showed complete recovery rate without residual impairment in 14% of patients with non-hemorrhagic stroke[90] and 25% in hemorrhagic stroke[91], respectively. In adult strokes, hemorrhagic stroke has higher mortality (23%) than non-hemorrhagic stroke[91].

In the long-term, cognitive impairment is significant in childhood stroke, and IQ (Intellectual Quotation) ranges widely and is lower than average[90, 92, 93]. As imagined, VIQ (Verbal IQ) is higher than PIQ (Performance IQ) in children with right hemisphere lesion, and PIQ is higher than VIQ in left hemisphere lesion[90, 93]. In spite of cognitive impairment, most of children return to mainstream school with/without support[57, 90]. Regardless of residual impairments and disabilities, they feel healthy and happy as normal children would[94].

General survival rate of pediatric stroke is better than adults[95, 96]. 5 year survival rate is 85%, and residual neurological deficits of 75% (hemiparesis, epilepsy, learning disabilities, visual field deficits, mental retardation)[97]. Idiopathic stroke have better prognosis than stroke associated with cardiac disease[98]. It is controversial but generally age is also an important prognostic factor[98]. The functional outcome of childhood stroke is more favorable than that of adult one. However, it is reported that infant stroke has poorer outcome than childhood stroke.

Poor outcome predictors are multiple cortical dysfunction, initial symptoms with altered level of consciousness with/without seizure, middle cerebral artery lesion, infant age onset, persistence of hemiparesis 1 month after stroke, and bilateral hemisphere lesions[57,90, 93,99, 100].

School re-entry is the final rehabilitation goal for children with stroke. A neuropsychological test including IQ indicates the details of the cognitive impairments. Based on the test results, school re-entry might be planned. Depending on medical conditions and the test results, home bound education, part time student, full time student, or classroom modification might be advised.

11. References

[1] Feign VL, Lawes CM, Bennett DA, Anderson CS. Stroke epidemiology: a review of population-based studies of incidence, prevalence, and case-fatality in the late 20th century. Lancet Neurol 2:43-53, 2003.

[2] Lauretani F, Saccavini M, Zaccaria B, Agosti M, Zampolini M, Franceschini M. Rehabilitation in patients affected by different types of stroke: A one-year follow-up study. Eur J Phys Rehabil Med 46(4):511-516, 2010.

[3] Shiber JR, Fontane E, Adewale A. Stroke registry: hemorrhaic vs ischemic strokes. Am J Emerg Med 28(3): 331-333, 2010.

[4] Wei JW, HeeleyEL, Wang J-G, Huang Y, Wong LKS, Li Z, Heritier S, Arima H, Anderson CS. Comparison of recovery patterns and prognostic indicators for ischemic and hemorrhagic stroke in China: the ChinaQUEST (Quality evaluation of stroke care and treatment) registry study. Stroke 41:1877-1883, 2010.

[5] Wardlaw JM, Murray V, Berge E, Del Zoppo GJ. Thrombolysis for acute ischemic stroke. Cochrane Database of Systematic Reviews (4):CD000213, 2009.

[6] Coughlan AK, Humprey M. Presenile stroke: long term outcome for patients and their families. Rheumatol Rehabil 21:115-120, 1982.

[7] Goto A, Okuda S, Ito S, Matsuoka Y, Ito E, Takahashi A, Sobue G. Locomotion outcome in hemiplegic patients with middle cerebral artery infarction: the difference between right- and left-sided lesions. J Stroke Cerebrovasc Dis 18(1):60-67, 2009.
[8] Fink JN, Frampton CM, Lyden P, Lees KR, Virtual International Stroke Trials Archives Investigators. Dose hemispheric lateralization influence functional and cardiovascular outcomes after stroke?: an analysis of placebo-treated patients from prospective acute stroke trials. Stroke 39(2):3335-3340, 2008.
[9] Howard G, Till JS, Toole JF, Matthews C, Truscott BL. Factors influencing return to work following cerebral infarction. JAMA 253(2):226-232, 1985.
[10] Mosch SC, Max JE, Tranel D. A matched lesion analysis of childhood versus adult-onset brain injury due to unilateral stroke. Cog Behav Neurol 18(1):5-17, 2005.
[11] Kwakkel G, Kollen BJ, van der Grond J, Prevo AJH. Probability of regaining dexterity in the flaccid upper extremity: impact of severity of paresis and time since onset in acute stroke. Stroke 34:2181-2186, 2003.
[12] Stone SP, Patel P, Greenwood RJ, Halligan PW. Measuring visual neglect in acute stroke and predicting its recovery: the visual neglect recovery index. J Neurol Neurosurg Psychiatry 55:431-436, 1992.
[13] Bowen A, McKenna K, Tallis R. Reasons for variability in the reported rate of occurrence of unilateral spatial neglect after stroke. Stroke 30:1196-1202, 1999.
[14] Katz N, Hartman-Maeir A, ring H, Soroker N. Functional disability and rehabilitation outcome in right hemisphere damage patients with and without unilateral spatial neglect. Arch Phys Med Rehabil 80:379-384, 1999.
[15] Buxbaum LJ, Ferraro MK, Veramonti T, Farne A, Whyte J, Ladavas E, Frassinetti F. Coslett HB. Hemispatial neglect: subtypes, neuroanatomy, and disability. Neurol 62:749-756, 2004.
[16] Jehkonen M, Ahonen J-P, Dastidar P, Koivisto A-M, Laippala P, Vilkki J, Molnar G, Predictors of discharge to home during the first year after right hemisphere stroke. Acta Neurol Scand 104:136-141, 2001.
[17] Jorgensen HS, Nakayama H, Raaschou HO, Olsen TS. Intracerebral hemorrhage versus infarction: stroke severity, risk factors, and prognosis. Ann Neurol 38(1):45-50, 1995.
[18] Leung AW, Cheng SK, Mak AK, Leung KK, Li LS, Lee TM. Functional gain in hemorrhagic stroke patients is predicted by functional level and cognitive abilities measured at hospital admission. Neurorehabil 27(4):351-358, 2010.
[19] Katrak PH, Black D, Peeva V. Do stroke patients with intracerebral hemorrhage have a better functional outcome than patients with cerebral infarction? PM&R 1:427-433, 2009.
[20] Paolucci S, Antonucci G, Grasso MG, Bragoni M, Coiro P. Functional outcome of ischemic and hemorrhagic stroke patients after inpatient rehabilitation: A matched comparison. Stroke 34:2861-2865, 2003.
[21] Chae J, Zorowitz RD, Johnston MV. Functional outcome of hemorrhagic and non-hemorrhagic stroke patients after in-patient rehabilitation. Am J Phys Med Rehabil 75:177-182, 1996.
[22] Franke CL, van Swieten JC, Algra A, van Gijin J. Prognostic factors in patients with intracerebral hematoma. J Neurol Neurosurg Psychiatry 55:653-657, 1992.

[23] Wei JW, Heeley EL, Wang JG, Huang Y, Wong LKS, Li Z, Heritier S, Arima H, Anderson CS. Comparison of recovery patterns and prognostic indicators for ischemic and hemorrhagic stroke in China: the ChinaQUEST(Quality evaluation of stroke care and treatment) registry study. Stroke 41:1877-1883, 2010.

[24] Toschke AM, Tilling K, Cox AM, Rudd AG. Heuschmann PU. Wolfe CD. Patient-specific recovery patterns over time measured by dependence in activities of daily living after stroke and post-stroke care: the South London Stroke Register (SLSR). Eur J Neurol 17:219-225, 2010.

[25] Daniel SK, Ballo LA, Mahoney M-C, Foundas AL. Clinical predictors of dysphagia and aspiration risk: outcome measures in acute stroke patients. Arch Phys Med Rehabil 81:1030-1033, 2000.

[26] Smithard DG, O'Neill PA, England RE, Park CL, Wyatt R, Martin DF, Morris J. The natural history of dysphagia following a stroke. Dysphagia 12(4):188-193, 1997.

[27] Meng N-H, Wang T-G, Lien I-N. Dysphagia in patients with brainstem stroke: incidence and outcome. Am J Phys Med Rehabil 79(2):170-175, 2000.

[28] Kovindha A, Wattanapan P, Dejpratham P, Permsirivanich W, Kuptniratsiku V. Prevalence of incontinence in patients after stroke during rehabilitation: a multi-center study. J Rehabil Med 41(6):489-491, 2009.

[29] Wilson D, Lowe E, Hoffman A, Rudd A, Wagg A. Urinary incontinence in stroke: results from the UK National Sentinel Audits of Stroke 1998-2004. Age & Ageing 37(5):542-546, 2008.

[30] Patel MD, Coshall C, Rudd AG, Wolfe CD. Cognition impairment after stroke: clinical determinants and its association with long-term stroke outcomes. J Am Geriatr Soc 50:700-709, 2002.

[31] Barker-Collo S, Feigin VL, Parag V, Lawes CM, Senior H. Neurol Auckland Stroke Outcome Study. Part2: cognition, and functional outcomes 5 years poststroke. Neurol 75(18):1608-1616, 2010

[32] Rojas-Fernandez CH, Moorhouse P. Current concepts in vascular cognitive impairment and pharmacotherapeutic implications. Ann Pharmocotherapy 43(7):1310-1323, 2009.

[33] Narasimhalu K, Effendy S, Sim CH, Lee JM, Chen I, Hia SB, Xue HL, Corrales MP, Chang HM, Wong MC, Chen CP, Tan EK. A randomized controlled trial of rivastigmine in patients with cognitive impairment no dementia because of cerebrovascular disease. Acta Neurol Scand 121(4):217- 224, 2010.

[34] Seniow J, Litwin M, Litwin T, Lesniak M, Czlonkowska A. New approach to the rehabilitation of post-stroke focal cognitive syndrome: effect of levedopa combined with speech and language therapy on functional recovery from aphasia. J Neurol Sci 283(1-2):214-218, 2009.

[35] Tobinick E. Rapid improvement of chronic stroke deficits after perispinal etanercept: three consecutive cases. CNS Drugs 25(2):145-155, 2011.

[36] Morris J. Effects of right hemisphere strokes on personality functioning. Topics Stroke Rehabil 16(6):425-430, 2009.

[37] Ayerbe L, Ayis S, Rudd AG, Heuschmann PU, Wolfe CD. Natural history, predictors, and association of depression 5 years after stroke: the South London Stroke Register. Stroke 42(7): 1907-1911, 2010.

[38] Ried LD, Jia H, Cameron R, Feng H, Wang X, Tueth M. Does prestroke depression impact poststroke depression and treatment? Am J Geriatr Psychiatry 18(7):624-633, 2010.

[39] Jorge RE, Starkstein SE. Robinson RG. Apathy following stoke. Canad J Psychiatry 55(6):350-354, 2010

[40] van Reekum R, Stuss DT, Ostrander L. Apathy:why care? J Neuropsychiatry Clin Neurosci 17:7-19, 2005.

[41] Long D, Young J, Dexamphetamine treatment in stroke. Q J Med 96:673-685, 2003

[42] Padala PR, Burke WJ, Bhatia SC, Petty F. Treatment of apathy with methylphenidate. J Neuropsychiatry Clin Neurosci 19:81-83, 2007.

[43] Spiegel DR, Kim J, Greene K, Conner C, Zamfir D. Apathy due to cerebrovascular accidents successfully treated with methylphenidate: a case series. J neuropsychiatry Clin Neurosci 21(2):216-219, 2009.

[44] Choi-Kwon S, Han SW, Kwon SU, Kang DW, Choi JM, Kim JS. Fluoxetine treatment in poststroke depression, emotional incontinence, and anger proneness: a double-bind , placebo-controlled study. Stroke 37(1):156-161, 2006.

[45] Robinson RG, Jorge RE, Clarence-Smith K. J Neuropsychiatry Clin Neurosci 20(2):178-84, 2008.

[46] Yamakawa Y, Satoh S, Sawa S, Ohta H, Asada T. Efficacy of milnacipran on poststroke depression on inpatient rehabilitation. J Psychiatry Clin Neurosci 59(6):705-710, 2005.

[47] Hackett ML, Anderson CS, House AO. Management of depression after stroke: a systematic review of pharmacological therapies. Stroke 36(5):1098-1103, 2005.

[48] Bowen A, Knapp P, Gillespie D, Nicholson DJ, Vail A. Non-pharmacological interventions for perceptual disorders following stroke and other adult-acquired, non-progressive brain injury. Cochrane Database of Systematic Reviews 4:CD007039, 2011.

[49] Jutai JW, Bhogal SK, Foley NC, Bayley M, Teasell RW, Speechley MR. Treatment of visual perceptual disorders post stroke. Topics Stroke Rehabil 10(2):77-106 , 2003.

[50] Tanei T, Kajita Y, Noda H, Takebayashi S, Nakatsubo D, Maesawa S, Wakabayashi T. Efficacy of motor cortex stimulation for intractable central neuropathic pain: comparison of stimulation parameters between post-stroke pain and other central pain. Neuro Medico-Chirug 51(1):8-14, 2011.

[51] McGeoch PD, Williams LE, Song T, Lee RR, Huang M, Ramachandran VS. Post-stroke tactile allodynia and its modulation by vestibular stimulation: a MEG case study. Acta Neurol Scand 119(6):404-409, 2009.

[52] McGeoch PD, Williams LE, Lee RR, Ramachandran VS. Behavioral evidence for vestibular stimulation as a treatment for central post-stroke pain. J Neurol Neurosurg Psychiatry 79(11):1298-1301, 2008.

[53] Pickering AE, Thornton SR, Love-Jones SJ, Steeds C, Patel NK. Analgesia in conjunction with normalization of thermal sensation following deep brain stimulation for central post-stroke pain. Pain 147(1-3):299-304, 2009.

[54] Twitchell TE. The restoration of motor function following hemiplegia in man. Brain 74:443-480, 1951.

[55] Hashimoto K, Higuchi K, Nakayama Y, Abo M. Ability for basic movement as an early predictor of functioning related to activities of daily living in stroke patients. Neurorehabil Neural Repair 21(4):353-357, 2007.

[56] Yamanaka T, Ishii M, Suzuki H. Short leg brace and stroke rehabilitation. Top Stroke Rehabil 11(3):3-5, 2004.

[57] Kim CT, Han J, Kim H. Pediatric stroke recovery: a descriptive analysis. Arch Phys Med Rehabil 90(4):657-662, 2009.

[58] Wandel A, Jorgensen HS, Nakayama H, Raaschou HO, Olsen TS. Prediction of walking function in stroke patients with initial lower extremity paralysis: the Copenhagen Stroke Study. Arch Phys Med Rehabil 81:736-738, 2000.

[59] Granger CV, Markello SJ, Graham JE, Deutsch A, Ottenbacher KJ. The Uniform Data System for Medical Rehabilitation: report of patients with stroke discharged from comprehensive medical programs in 2000-2007. Am J Phys Med Rehabil 88:961-972, 2009.

[60] Ottenbacher KJ, Smith PM, Illig SB, et al. Trends in length of stay, living setting, functional outcome, and mortality following medical rehabilitation. JAMA 292:1687-1695, 2004.

[61] Duarte E, Marco E, Muniesa JM, Belmonte R, Aguilar JJ, Escalada F. Early detection of non-ambulatory survivors six months after stroke. Neurorehabil 26(4):317-323, 2010.

[62] Kollen B, van de Port I, Lindeman E, Twisk J, Kwakkel G. Predicting improvement in gait after stroke: a longitudinal prospective study. Stroke 36(12):2676-2680, 2005.

[63] Frech B, Thomas LH, Leathley MJ, Sutton CJ, McAdam J, Forster A. Langhorne P, Price CI, Walker A, Watkins CL. Repetitive task training for improving functional ability after stroke. Cochrane Database Syst Rev 17(4):CD006073, 2007.

[64] Taub E, Miller NE, Novack TA, Cook III EW, Fleming WC, Nepomuceno CS, Connell JS, Crago JE. Technique to improve chronic motor deficit after stroke. Arch Phys Med Rehabil 74:347-354, 1993.

[65] Wolf SL, Winstein CJ, Miller JP, Taub E, Uswate G, Morris D, Giuliani C, Light KE, Nicholas-Larsen D: EXCITE investigators. Effect of constraint-induced movement therapy on upper extremity function 3 to 9 months after stroke: the EXCITE randomized clinical trial. JAMA 296(17):2095-2104, 2006.

[66] Wolf SL, Thompson PA, Winstein CJ, Miller JP, Blanton SR, Nicholas-Larsen D, Morris D, Uswate G, Taub E, Light KE, Sawaki L. The EXCITE stroke trial: comparing early and delayed constraint-induced movement therapy. Stroke 41(10):2309-2315, 2010.

[67] Corbetta D, Sirtori V, Moja L, Gatti R. Constrained-induced movement therapy in storke patients: systematic review and meta-analysis. Europ J Physical Med & Rehabil 46(4):537-544, 2010.

[68] Dromerick AW, Lang CE, Birkenmeier RL, Wagner JM, Miller JP, Videen TO, Powers WJ, Wolf SL, and Edwards DF. Very early constraint-induced movement during stroke rehabilitation (VECTORS): a single-center RCT. Neurol 73:195-201, 2009.

[69] Lum PS, Burgar CG, Shor PC, et al. Robot-assisted movement training compared with conventional therapy techniques for the rehabilitation of upper-limb motor function after stroke. Arch Phys Med Rehabil 83(7): 952-959, 2002.

[70] Takahashi CD, Der-Yeghiaian L, Motiwala RR, Cramer SC. Robot-based hand motor therapy after stroke. Brain 131:425-437, 2008.

[71] Volpe BT, Krebs HI, Hogan N, Edelstein L, Diels C, Aisen M. A novel approach to stroke rehabilitation. Robot-aided sensorimotor stimulation. Neurol 54(10):1938-1944, 2000.

[72] Lo AC, Guarino PD, Richards LG, et al. Robot-assisted therapy for long-term upper-limb impairment after stroke. N Eng J Med 362:1772-1783, 2010.

[73] Krebs HI, Ferraro M, Buerger SP, Newbery MJ, Makiyama A, Sandmann M, Lynch D, Volpe BT, Hogan N. Rehabilitation robotics: pilot trial of spatial extension for MIT-Manus. J Neuroengineer Rehabil1:5-19, 2004.

[74] Buch E, Weber C, Cohen LG, Braun C, Dimyan MA, Ard T, Mellinger J, Caria A, Soekadar S, Fourkas A, Birbaumer N. Think to move: a neuromagnetic brain-computer interface (BCI) system for chronic stroke. Stroke 39(3):910-917, 2008.

[75] Broetz D, Braun C, Weber C, Soekadar SR, Caria A, Birbaumer N. Combination of brain-computer interface training and goal-directed physical therapy in chronic stroke: a case study. Neurorehabil Neural Repair 24(7):674-679, 2010.

[76] Bradberry TJ, Gentili RJ, Contreras-Vidal JL. Reconstructing three-dimensional hand movements from noninvasive electroencephalographic signals. J Neurosci 30(9):3432-3437, 2010.

[77] Saposnik G, Levin M. Outcome Research Canada (SORCan) Working Group. Virtual reality in stroke rehabilitation: a meta-analysis and implications for clinicians. Stroke 42(5):1380-1386, 2011.

[78] Henderson AH. Virtual reality in stroke rehab: a systematic review for upper motor recovery. Top Stroke Rehabil 14(2):52-61, 2007.

[79] Jorgensen HS, Reith H, Nakayama H, Kammersgaard LP, Raaschou H, Olsen TS. What determines good recovery in patients with the most severe stroke. The Copenhagen Stroke Study. Stroke 30:2008-2012, 1999.

[80] Al-Eithan MH, Amin M, Robert AA) The effect of hemiplegia/hemiparesis, diabetes, and hyperteniosn on hospital length of stay after stroke. Neurosci 16(3):253-256, 2011.

[81] Lynch JK, Hirtz DG, DeVeber G, Nelson KB. Report of the National Institute of Neurological Disorders and Stroke workshop on perinatal and childhood stroke. Pediatr 109:116-123, 2002.

[82] deVeber G. Roach ES, Riela AR, Wiznitzer. Stroke in children: recognition, treatment, and future directions. Sem Pediatr Neurol 7(4):309-317, 2000.

[83] Giroud M, Lemesele M, Gouyon JB, Nivelon JL, Milan C, Dumas R. Cerebrovascular disease in children under 16 years of age in the city of Dijion, France: a study of incidence and clinical features from 1985 to 1993, J Clin Epidemiol 48:1343-1348, 1995.

[84] Christerson S, Stromber B. Childhood stroke in Sweden 1: incidence, symptoms, risk factors, and short-term outcome. Acta Paediatr Scand 99:1641-1649, 2010.

[85] Yock-Corrales A, Mackay MT, Mosley I, Maixner W, Baabl FE, Acute childhood arterial ischemic and hemorrhagic stroke in the emergency department. Ann Em Med 58(2):156-163, 2011.

[86] Nelson KB, Dambrosia JM, Grether JK, Phillips TM. Neonatal cytokines and coagulation factors in children with cerebral palsy. Ann Neurol 44:665-675, 1998.

[87] Dizon-Townson D, Miller C, Sibai B, Spong CY, Thom E, Wendel G Jr, Wensgtrom K, Samuels P, Cotroneo MA, Moawad A, Sorokin Y, Meis P, Miodovnik M, O'Sullivan MJ, Conway D, Wapner RJ, Gabbe SG. The relationship of the factor V Leiden mutation and pregnancy outcome s for mother and fetus. Obste Gynecol 106(3):517-524, 2005.

[88] Gadian DG, Issacs EB, Cross JH, Connelly A, Jackson GD, King MD, Neville BG, Vargha-Khadem F. Lateralization of brain function in childhood revealed by magnetic resonance spectroscopy. Neurol 46(4):974-977, 1996.

[89] Vicari S, Stiles J, Stern C, Resca A. Spatial grouping activity in children with early cortical and subcortical lesion. Dev Med Child Neurol 40(2):90-94, 1998.

[90] Ganesan V, Hogan A, Shack N, Gordon A, Issacs E, Kirkham FJ. Outcome after ischemic stroke in childhood. Develop Med Child Neurol 42(7):455-461, 2000.

[91] Blom I, De Schryver EL, Kappelle LJ, Rinkel GJ, Jennekens-Schinkel A, Peters AC. Prognosis of haemorrhagic stroke in childhood: a long-term follow-up study. Dev Med Child Neurol 45:233-239, 2003.

[92] Steinlin M, Roellin K, Schroth G. long-term follow-up after stroke in childhood. Eur J Pediatr 163:245-250, 2004.

[93] Kolk A, Talvik T. Cognitive outcome of children with early-onset hemiparesis. J Child Neurol 15(9):581-587, 2000.

[94] De Schryver EL, Kappelle LJ, Jennekens-Schinkel A, Boudewyn Peters AC. Prognosis of ischemic stroke in childhood: a long-term follow-up study. Dev Med Child Neurol 42(5):313-318, 2000.

[95] Giroud M, Lemesele M, Madinier G, Manceau E, Osseby GV, Dumas R. Stroke in children under 16 years of age. Clinical and etiological difference with adults. Acta Neurol Scand 96(6):401-406, 1997.

[96] Kleinman JT, gailloud P, Jordan LC. Recovery from spatial neglect and hemiplegia in a child despite a large anterior circulation stroke and Wallerian degeneration. J Child Neurol 25(4):500-503, 2010.

[97] Schoenberg BS, Mellinger JF, Schoenberg DG. Cerebrovascular disease in infants and children: a study of incidence, clinical features, and survival. Neurol 28(8):763-768, 1978.

[98] Dusser A, Goutieres F, Aicardi J. Ischemic strokes in children. J Child Neurol 1(2):131-136, 1986.

[99] Delsing BJ, Catsman-Berrevoets CE, Appel IM. Early prognostic indicators of outcome in ischemic childhood stroke. Pediatr Neurol 24(4):283-289, 2001.

[100] Abram HS, Knepper LE, Warty VS, Painter MJ. Natural history, prognosis, and lipid abnormalities of idiopathic ischemic childhood stroke. J Child Neurol 11(4):276-282, 1996.

3

Myotonometric Measurement of Muscular Properties of Hemiparetic Arms in Stroke Patients

Li-Ling Chuang[1], Ching-Yi Wu[2] and Keh-Chung Lin[1]
[1]*National Taiwan University, Taipei,*
[2]*Chang Gung University, Taoyuan,*
Taiwan

1. Introduction

Stroke is the leading cause of functional disability. The most significant impairment developed in individuals with stroke is the loss of normal skeletal muscle tone on the affected side, which leads to the lack of normal, controlled movements and further limits the individual's ability to carry out tasks of daily living. Session 1 of this chapter describes skeletal muscle changes after stroke and defines functional roles of muscle tone, elasticity, and stiffness. Session 2 discusses methods for measuring muscle tone, elasticity, and stiffness, including common clinical measure, laboratory measure, and a new novel myotonometer. Session 3 presents metric properties of the myotonometric measurements in previous studies. Session 4 provides an overview of myotonometric measurement relevant to stroke motor rehabilitation and future research directions, with special attention on the reliability, validity, and sensitivity to treatment-induced change of using the myotonometer to measure muscle properties of relaxed extensor digitorum, flexor carpi radialis, and flexor carpi ulnaris muscles in patients with stroke. Session 5 concludes the clinical value of myotonometric measurements in stroke rehabilitation.

1.1 The definition and functional role of muscle tone, elasticity, and stiffness

Muscle tone involves active tension and passive (resting) intrinsic viscoelastic tone (Ditroilo et al., 2011; Masi & Hannon, 2008; Simons & Mense, 1998). Human resting muscle tone was defined as the passive tonus or tension of skeletal muscle that derives from its intrinsic molecular viscoelastic properties (Masi & Hannon, 2008); that is, resting muscle tone is the viscoelastic stiffness without contractile activity (Simons & Mense, 1998). The functional roles of passive muscle tone are for maintaining balanced stability posture and for achieving energy-efficient costs for prolonged duration without fatigue (Masi & Hannon, 2008).

Muscle elasticity is defined as the property of a muscle to return to its original form or shape after removing a deforming force, and muscle stiffness is a muscle's resistance to deformation (Masi & Hannon, 2008; Panjabi, 1992; Simons & Mense, 1998). Factors that affect resting muscle tone, elasticity, and stiffness include neuromuscular disorders (Alhusaini et al., 2010; Hafer-Macko et al., 2008; Ratsep & Asser, 2011), massage (Huang et al., 2010), stretching maneuvers (Magnusson, 1998; Reisman et al., 2009), aerobic exercise (Hafer-Macko et al., 2008), the length of skeletal muscle (Ditroilo et al., 2011; Hoang et al., 2007), and eccentric exercise (Hoang et al., 2007; Whitehead et al., 2001). Decreased muscle elasticity brings on easier fatigueability and limited movement speed (Gapeyeva & Vain, 2008). Muscle performing the movement (agonist) stretches out the antagonist muscle. Antagonist muscles with higher stiffness require greater effort for stretching, which leads to worse economy of movement (Gapeyeva & Vain, 2008).

1.2 Skeletal muscle changes after hemiparetic stroke

Evidence has revealed that the mechanisms of abnormal muscle tone in stroke patients include physiologic as well as mechanical (viscoelastic) properties of muscle (Dietz et al., 1981; Katz & Rymer, 1989; Pandyan et al., 1999; Rydahl & Brouwer, 2004). Significant changes in structural and mechanical properties of the paralyzed muscle occur after a stroke (Sjostrom et al., 1980; Svantesson et al., 2000). Muscular atrophy and muscle phenotype shift to fast-twitch fiber proportions in the hemiparetic leg muscle after a stroke and relate to muscle fatigue, poor fitness, poor physical performance, and neurologic gait deficit (Hafer-Macko et al., 2008). Spasticity (hyperactivity of stretch reflexes) and hypertonia (i.e., increased stiffness and viscosity) are common impairments after stroke (de Vlugt et al., 2010; Katz & Rymer, 1989). Spasticity is attributed to increased muscle tone related to hyperreflexia according to Lance (1980) who defined spasticity as a velocity-dependent increase in tonic stretch reflexes (muscle tone) with exaggerated tendon jerks, resulting from reflex hyperexcitability (Lance, 1980). Hypertonia, i.e., increased resistance to passive stretch, was more associated with intrinsic changes of the muscles than increased reflex activity (O'Dwyer et al., 1996). Moreover, the muscle stiffness of the affected leg was much higher than that of the contralateral leg after a stroke, suggesting a difference in the passive mechanical properties of the muscles of the spastic limb compared with the normal limb (Svantesson et al., 2000).

2. Methods for measuring muscle tone, elasticity, and stiffness

In recent decades, new methods, such as botulinum toxin, have been increasingly used to treat spasticity due to stroke (Shaw et al., 2011). Thus, the need for a quantitative measurement of muscle tone in the clinical setting has been highlighted. The development of an adequate tool that is reliable, valid, and responsive to measure the progression of muscle properties and success of treatments becomes urgent (Haas & Crow, 1995).

2.1 Common clinical measure of muscle tone

The Ashworth Scale (AS) and the Modified Ashworth Scale (MAS) are the most common clinical measures of muscle tone, rating the resistance perceived to passive stretch of the muscle with a 5- or 6-point ordinal scale, respectively (Ashworth, 1964; Bohannon & Smith, 1987; Pandyan et al., 1999). Although they are useful in the clinic, these two measures have been criticized for:

- not standardizing stretch velocity in manual testing (de Vlugt et al., 2010),
- not quantifying resistance in absolute units (Pandyan et al., 1999),
- not providing an assessment of activated muscle tone (Sommerfeld et al., 2004),

- subjectively grading and clustering of scores (Katz & Rymer, 1989; Pandyan et al., 1999),
- only being applicable for the extremities (Leonard et al., 2001),
- lacking sensitivity for detecting smaller degrees of changes in spasticity (Lance, 1980),
- poor discrimination between increased muscle tone and soft-tissue stiffness (de Vlugt et al., 2010; Sheean & McGuire, 2009), and
- lacking correlation with functional changes after treatment (Ward, 2000).

The reliability and validity of both scales have also been questioned (Aarrestad et al., 2004; Katz & Rymer, 1989; Leonard et al., 2003; Pandyan et al., 1999; Pomeroy et al., 2000).

The AS has only been validated for measuring spasticity around the elbow after stroke (Lee et al., 1989). The MAS is reliable for measuring muscle tone in certain muscle groups, such as the elbow, wrist, and knee flexors, in stroke patients (Gregson et al., 2000). These critiques and limitations reaffirm the need for identifying suitable clinical tools that reliably and accurately assess the biomechanical properties of muscle, including tone, elasticity, and stiffness (Pandyan et al., 1999).

2.2 Laboratory measure of mechanical properties of muscle

The mechanical properties of muscle are generally assessed in laboratories with expensive and heavy equipment, such as isokinetic and ultrasound machines (Ditroilo et al., 2011). Ultrasonography is limited to superficial structures and does not assess specific muscle mechanical properties (Nordez et al., 2008).

2.3 A new novel instrument for measuring muscle tone, elasticity, and stiffness simultaneously

For clinical applications, mechanical properties, such as muscle elasticity and stiffness, may not be accurately estimated by the clinical scales. A novel hand-held myotonometer, the Myoton myometer (Müomeetria AS, Tallinn, Estonia) device, provides painless and noninvasive means to obtain quantitative and objective assessments of mechanical properties of muscles (Gapeyeva & Vain, 2008; Roja et al., 2006). The Myoton myometer was primarily developed for testing the superficial skeletal muscles (Gapeyeva & Vain, 2008). The principal differences between myotonometry and traditional measures of muscle tone are that the former measures the tone, elasticity, and stiffness simultaneously and quantitatively (Gapeyeva & Vain, 2008), is not affected by tester strength (Leonard et al., 2003), and is more sensitive to detect small changes (Aarrestad et al., 2004; Leonard et al., 2001). The myotonometer has the additional advantages of an appropriate size for being portable, relatively inexpensive and convenient to use, and relatively easy to administer over a wide range of postural or extremity musculature (Aarrestad et al., 2004; Ditroilo et al., 2011; Gapeyeva & Vain, 2008; Gubler-Hanna et al., 2007; Ianieri et al., 2009).

Muscle properties can be measured with the myotonometer without the muscle being moved, which might be helpful with patients who have limited range of motion or pain with movement (Leonard et al., 2003). Its application leads to a more objective assessment of numeric parameters of muscle tone, elasticity, and stiffness within minutes (Aarrestad et al., 2004). Therefore, the myotonometer appears to be clinically applicable without compromising the precision related to more complex laboratory methods and ensures a better pathophysiologic vision of all three muscle properties.

From discerning muscular properties using myotonometric measurements, clinicians would be able to have a better understanding of the pathologic processes of muscle functions in individuals with spastic muscle secondary to stroke, design a specific rehabilitation program for each patient, make appropriate clinical decision, plan a more targeted and customized treatment specifically for each patient with abnormal muscle properties, and assess the efficacy of specific therapeutic treatment (Pandyan et al., 1999; Wade, 1992). This chapter will illustrate the metric properties of myotonometric measurement based on previous studies and our recent research in stroke rehabilitation.

3. Metric properties of the myotonometric measurements: Reliability and validity

Metric properties of the myotonometric measurements, such as reliability, validity, and responsiveness are the prerequisites of a useful measurement. From literature review, previous studies focused on examining reliability and validity of myotonometric measurement. The results of previous reliability studies have indicated that myotonometry is highly reliable for measuring skeletal muscle viscoelastic parameters in healthy individuals (Bizzini & Mannion, 2003; Ditroilo et al., 2011; Gavronski et al., 2007; Leonard et al., 2004; Leonard et al., 2003; Viir et al., 2006), children with cerebral palsy (Aarrestad et al., 2004; Lidstrom et al., 2009), and patients with Parkinson's disease (Marusiak et al., 2010; Ratsep & Asser, 2011). There is no study investigating the reliability of the myotonometer in stroke patients, which may limit the interpretation of the change for myotonometric measurements.

The construct validity of the myotonometer has been established in healthy individuals (Gubler-Hanna et al., 2007), patients with upper motor neuronal disorders (Leonard et al., 2001), and stroke survivors (Rydahl & Brouwer, 2004). Studies have shown that muscle stiffness increased with increasing contractile force and muscle activation, indicating that muscle stiffness during contracted conditions provides an indirect measure of muscle strength (Aarrestad et al., 2004; Bizzini & Mannion, 2003; Gubler-Hanna et al., 2007; Leonard et al., 2001; Rydahl & Brouwer, 2004). Moreover, Katz and Rymer (1989) demonstrated that extending a limb against passive resistance may be more related to the viscoelastic properties of the soft tissues than to spasticity, indicating that biomechanical measures correlate most closely with motor function. These findings provide the theoretic basis for use of muscle strength and motor function measures to further validate myotonometric measures.

4. Metric properties of the myotonometric measurements: Reliability, validity, and responsiveness of the Myoton-3 myometer in patients with stroke

Previous metric studies of myotonometry have not yet reported the responsiveness. The responsiveness of the instrument is its ability to detect change over time, which is an important quality to detect small changes in muscle properties and assess the effectiveness of specific treatment. Additionally, previous reliability and validity studies applied the myotonometer on large muscles of the trunk and extremities. Wrist and finger control is the motor function most likely to be impaired after stroke. Proper function of the muscles involved in hand movements is crucial to manual exploration and manipulation of the environment.

Our recent study (Chuang et al., 2012) addressed the test-retest reliability, validity, and responsiveness of the Myoton-3 myometer used for assessing tone, elasticity, and stiffness of the affected forearm muscles under a relaxed state in stroke rehabilitation. The Myoton-3 myometer represents a new technology to quantify mechanical properties of resting and contractiling muscles. To the best of our knowledge, this was the first report to show the metric soundness of the Myoton-3 myometer for assessing muscle tone, elasticity, and stiffness of the extensor digitorum, flexor carpi radialis, and flexor carpi ulnaris muscles in patients with stroke. Information reported in this study that is relevant to purposes of this book chapter is summarized below.

4.1 Study sample

We recruited 67 patients (40 men and 27 women) who were a mean age of 54.67 (SD, 10.90) years. The mean time since the stroke onset was 21.12 (SD, 13.63) months, and 31 patients had left hemiplegia. All participants had sustained a first-ever stroke, Brunnstrom stage III to V for the proximal and distal upper extremity (UE) (Brunnstrom, 1970), MAS ≤ 2 in any joint of the UE (Bohannon & Smith, 1987), no cognitive impairment (Mini-Mental State Examination score ≥ 24) (Folstein et al., 1975), not participated in any experimental rehabilitation or drug studies, and not used anti-spasticity drugs for the UE musculature (e.g., botulinum toxin type A) during the study period. Institutional Review Board approval was obtained from the study sites, and written informed consent was obtained from each patient before inclusion.

4.2 Instrument

The functional state of the participants' skeletal muscles was assessed by using myotonometric measurements with the Myoton-3 myometer, created at the University of Tartu in Estonia (Vain, 1995).

The Myoton-3 myometer has a two-armed lever. On the long lever is the testing end and on the short lever is the core of the electromagnet. The essence of the method lies in giving the muscle a short mechanical impulse to evoke decaying oscillations of the muscle because of the elastic behavior of the muscle. The working principles of the Myoton-3 myometer were as follows: the testing end of the Myoton-3 was placed perpendicular to the skin surface above the muscle to be measured and a brief mechanical impulse was applied, shortly followed by a quick release to the muscle through an acceleration probe. The characteristics of the muscle deformation and also the damped oscillations of the muscle evoked after the quick release of the testing end were recorded by the acceleration transducer at the testing end of the device. At the moment the Myoton-3 myometer pickup has created the maximum compression of the tested muscle, the corresponding acceleration a_{max} characterizes the resistance force of the muscle for the deformation depth Δl (Figure 1).

The parameters of the graph characterize the functional state of the muscle. Displacement (s) is the difference in the initial position of the tested muscle and its final position. The relationships between position, velocity, and acceleration form an important application of the definite derivative. The velocity is defined by the derivative of position at a given time; whereas the acceleration is defined by the derivative of velocity at a given time. The average velocity of the muscle is the total displacement during an extended period of time, divided by that period of time. Average acceleration is the total change in velocity over an extended period of time, divided by the duration of that period. In Figure 1, time moment 1 (t_1) denotes the beginning of the mechanical impulse to the muscle. The maximum of the deformation speed is obtained at time moment 3 (t_3) and from that moment the muscle deformation speed decreases and at time moment 4 (t_4) the acceleration transducer of the device has reached the maximum depth of its trajectory inward the muscle. At time moment 5 (t_5) the forces of muscle elasticity have given to the transducer its maximum speed upwards. At time moment 6 (t_6) this speed has decreased to zero under the influence of gravity. The above-described process repeats itself until the oscillation has decayed completely.

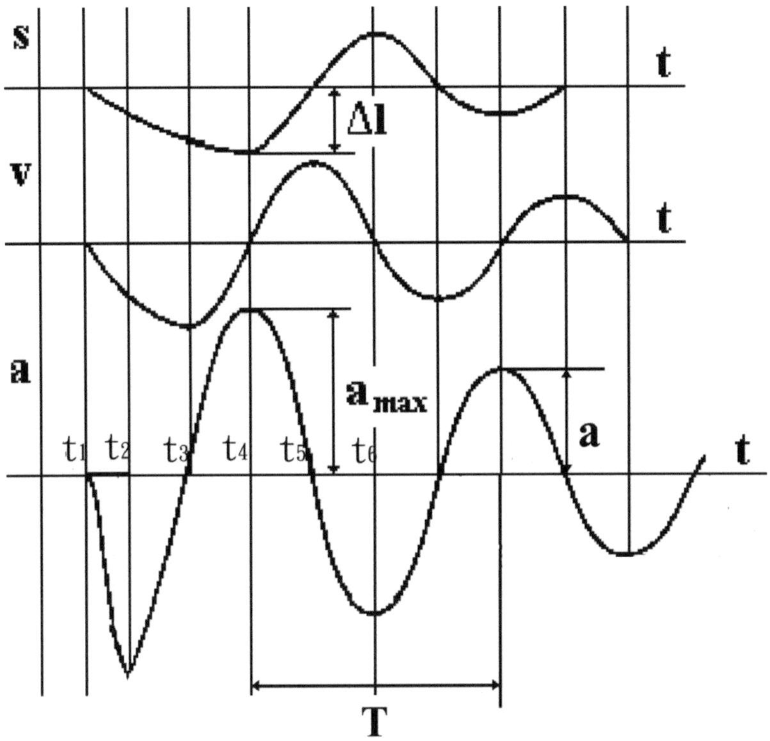

Fig. 1. An oscillation graph of the muscle shows the acceleration (a), velocity (v), and displacement (s) of the muscle produced in the process of damped natural oscillation measured by the Myoton-3 myometer.

The parameters measured by the myotonometer are oscillation frequency, decrement, and stiffness. The acceleration value of the first period of oscillations characterizes the deformation of the muscle, and the value of the next oscillation period provides the basis for calculating the oscillation frequency (Hz). The oscillation frequency is usually 11 to 16 Hz in relaxation and 18 to 40 Hz in contraction, depending on the muscle (Gapeyeva & Vain, 2008). The frequency of the damped oscillations characterizes the muscle tone, the mechanical tension in a relaxed muscle. The higher the value, the more tense is the muscle. The frequency of the damping was calculated as:

$$\text{Frequency (Hz)} = 1 / T$$

where T is the oscillation period in seconds (Figure 1).

The logarithmic decrement of the damping oscillations characterizes muscle elasticity, which is the ability of the muscle to restore its initial shape after contraction. Elasticity is inversely proportional to the decrement. If the decrement of trained muscles decreases, the muscle elasticity increases. The decrement values are usually 1.0 to 1.2, depending on the muscle. The logarithmic decrement of damping was calculated as:

$$\text{Decrement} = \ln (a_{max} / a)$$

where a_{max} is the maximal amplitude of oscillation and a is the oscillation amplitude (Figure 1).

Stiffness (N/m) reflects the resistance of the muscle to the force deforming the muscle (Roja et al., 2006). The usual range of stiffness values is 150 to 300 N/m for resting muscle and may exceed 1000 N/m for contracted muscles (Gapeyeva & Vain, 2008). Stiffness was calculated as a ratio between the force applied and the muscle deformation:

$$\text{Stiffness (N/m)} = f / \Delta l = m \times a_{max} / \Delta l$$

where f is the force applied, m is the mass of the testing end (kg), a_{max} is the maximal acceleration of oscillation (meter/second^2), and Δl is the deformation depth of the muscle (meter) (Figure 1).

4.3 Procedures

Myotonometric testing of the affected extensor digitorum, the flexor carpi radialis, and the flexor carpi ulnaris in relaxed state was conducted before and after treatments. All participants received a 1.5-hour therapy session 5 times per week for 4 weeks. A senior occupational therapist administered the outcome measures at baseline and after the 4-week treatment. Before measurement, participants were informed about standard measurement procedure with their elbow flexion 30° to 45°, the palm downward for the affected extensor digitorum measurement and palm upward for measurements of the affected flexor carpi radialis and ulnaris muscles (Figure 2) (Gapeyeva & Vain, 2008). The investigator applied resistance to the tested muscles and requested participants to make an effort to resist. At the same time, the investigator established the location of the tested muscles by the visual-palpatory test. Participants were instructed to lie supine and relax the muscles maximally. Three trials were recorded with a 1-second interval, and the average value was used for analysis. To investigate test-retest reliability, 58 of the 67 individuals were tested twice on the affected side with the same procedure, 30 minutes apart, at baseline.

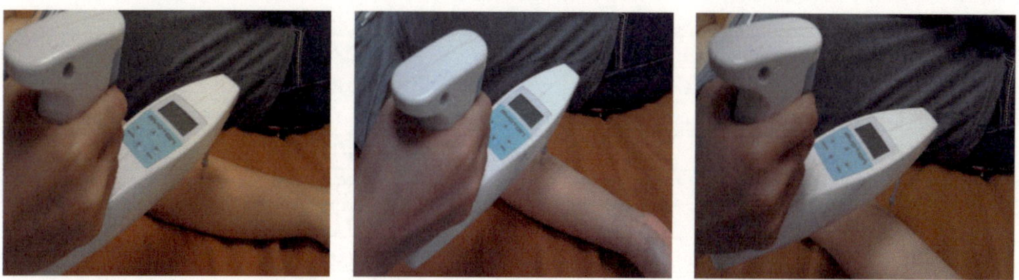

(A) (B) (C)

Fig. 2. The standard measurement location of the measured muscles: (A) extensor digitorum, (B) flexor carpi radialis, and (C) flexor carpi ulnaris

4.4 Criterion measures

The Myoton-3 measures, as well as criterion measures for hand strength, including grip strength, lateral pinch power, and palmar pinch power, the Action Research Arm Test (ARAT), and Brunnstrom stage were performed before and after treatments.

4.5 Data analysis

Statistical analyses were performed with SPSS version 16.0 software (SPSS Inc, Chicago, IL USA) and values of $P < 0.05$ were considered statistically significant. The analysis of variance (ANOVA) was used to compare the baseline and posttreatment characteristics of the 3 affected muscles. The Bonferroni method was used for post hoc pairwise comparisons.

Test-retest reliability of the Myoton-3 was determined by using the intraclass correlation coefficient (ICC) with 95% confidence intervals (CIs); an ICC value exceeding 0.80 indicated high reliability (Weir, 2005).

Concurrent validity of the Myoton-3 was determined using the Pearson correlation (r) test to establish relationships with hand strength and the Spearman rho (ρ) test to calculate the degree of correlations with the ARAT and Brunnstrom stage, respectively. The strength of correlations was interpreted as low (0.00-0.25), fair (0.25-0.50), moderate to good (0.50-0.75), and good to excellent (>0.75) (Portney, 2009).

The standardized response mean (SRM) was used as the index of the responsiveness of the Myoton-3 according to changes of the affected and unaffected limbs from pretreatment to postest. The SRM was estimated as the ratio of the mean change scores to the standard deviation of the change scores from patients whose myotonometric measures improved over time (i.e., the change score from pretreatment to posttreatment was negative in muscle properties), and the values were categorized as large (>0.8), moderate (0.5-0.8), and small (0.2-0.5) (Cohen, 1988).

4.6 Results

4.6.1 Comparison of the muscular properties of the extensor digitorum, flexor carpi radialis, and flexor carpi ulnaris at pretreatment and posttreatment

Table 1 summarizes the mean (SD) of the myotonometric measurements for muscle tone, elasticity, and stiffness of the extensor digitorum, flexor carpi radialis, and flexor carpi ulnaris muscles at pretreatment and posttreatment.

	Muscular properties	Extensor digitorum	Flexor carpi radialis	Flexor carpi ulnaris
Pretreatment Mean (SD)	Tone (Hz)	17.60 (2.82)	14.78 (3.01)	13.45 (2.80)
	Elasticity	1.89 (0.27)	1.31 (0.31)	1.35 (0.33)
	Stiffness (N/m)	354.90 (62.16)	297.85 (65.47)	272.85 (57.72)
Posttreatment Mean (SD)	Tone (Hz)	17.03 (2.64)	15.03 (3.19)	13.39 (2.40)
	Elasticity	1.84 (0.34)	1.31 (0.40)	1.40 (0.34)
	Stiffness (N/m)	341.24 (51.02)	309.26 (74.09)	268.94 (55.05)

Table 1. Mean and standard deviation of the myotonometric measurements for muscular properties of the 3 affected forearm muscles

Results of the ANOVA showed a significant difference in muscle tone, elasticity, and stiffness among the 3 affected muscles before and after treatment ($P < 0.0001$). Post hoc analyses revealed that muscle tone and stiffness of the extensor digitorum were significantly higher than those of the flexor carpi radialis and flexor carpi ulnaris at both pretreatment and posttreatment (pretreatment tone and stiffness: $P < 0.0001$, posttreatment tone: $P < 0.0001$, posttreatment stiffness: $P = 0.008$, $P < 0.0001$, resepctively). Muscle tone of the flexor carpi radialis was significantly higher than that of flexor carpi ulnaris at pretreatment and posttreatment ($P = 0.025$, 0.002, respectively). Muscle stiffness of the flexor carpi radialis was significantly higher than that of flexor carpi ulnaris at posttreatment ($P = 0.001$). Muscle elasticity of the extensor digitorum was significantly lower than the elasticity of flexor carpi radialis and flexor carpi ulnaris at both pretreatment and posttreatment ($P< 0.0001$, $P< 0.0001$, respectively). In general, the extensor digitorum showed higher tone and stiffness with lower elasticity compared to the flexor carpi radialis and ulnaris muscles.

4.6.2 Reliability of the Myoton-3 myometer in patients with stroke

The test-retest reliability was performed on a subset of 58 participants who underwent two pretreatment measurements. The Myoton-3 myometer showed high to very high test-retest reliability for muscle properties in affected extensor digitorum, flexor carpi radialis, and flexor carpi ulnaris (ICC, 0.86-0.96).

Our study indicated that the Myoton-3 is a highly reliable measurement tool with high test-retest reliability under relaxed conditions in measurements of affected forearm muscles of stroke patients. These findings are similar to those reported of the myotonometer for different muscles and study populations. The reliability of the myotonometer was high in the biceps brachii, rectus femoris, biceps femoris, and gastrocnemius in healthy individuals (Bizzini & Mannion, 2003; Ditroilo et al., 2011; Leonard et al., 2003; Marusiak et al., 2010); the biceps brachii in patients with Parkinson's disease (Marusiak et al., 2010); and in the brachii, gastrocnemius, and rectus femoris in children with cerebral palsy (Aarrestad et al., 2004; Lidstrom et al., 2009). In general, the Myoton-3 myometer is reliable for measurements in healthy individuals as well as for various patient populations.

4.6.3 Validity of the Myoton-3 myometer in patients with stroke

Significant correlations existed between the tone and stiffness of the 3 muscles and palmar pinch strength, between those of the flexor carpi radialis & ulnaris muscles and lateral pinch strength, and between those of the flexor carpi radialis and the ARAT at posttreatment. The posttreatment elasticity of the two flexor carpi muscles was significantly correlated with grip strength. The pretreatment elasticity of the flexor carpi ulnaris was significantly correlated with posttreatment grip strength, and the pretreatment muscle tone and stiffness of the flexor carpi radialis were significantly correlated with palmar pinch strength and ARAT. There was no significant correlations existed between the Brunnstrom stage and muscle properties of the 3 muscles at pretreatment. Posttreatment extensor digitorum tone and flexor carpi radialis stiffness were significantly correlated with the Brunnstrom stage.

The results of the concurrent validity showed partly significant associations between forearm muscle properties and hand strength and UE motor function, especially at posttreatment, which indicates that they might measure similar constructs. Our present findings were compatible with those from a previous study reporting a correlation between muscle stiffness and muscle strength of the quadriceps (Bizzini & Mannion, 2003). In this study, the elasticity of the two wrist flexors tended to increase with greater grip strength at posttreatment. At posttreatment, the elasticity of the extensor digitorum and muscle tone and stiffness of the two wrist flexors tended to increase with greater lateral pinch strength. The muscle tone and stiffness of the extensor digitorum and the two wrist flexors appeared to increase with greater palmar pinch strength. The pretreatment and posttreatment muscle tone and stiffness of the flexor carpi radialis were correlated to palmar pinch strength and ARAT.

4.6.4 Responsiveness of the Myoton-3 myometer in patients with stroke receiving rehabilitation

The responsiveness of the extensor digitorum was higher than those of the flexor carpi radialis and ulnaris, with moderate to high for the affected extensor digitorum and small to moderate for the affected flexor carpi radialis and ulnaris. The responsiveness of the muscle tone and elasticity was moderate for the affected extensor digitorum and small for the affected flexor carpi radialis and ulnaris (tone: -0.57 vs -0.39 vs -0.35; elasticity: -0.75 vs -0.44 vs -0.31). The responsiveness of the elasticity of the affected extensor digitorum was significantly higher than that of the affected flexor carpi ulnaris (difference in SRM, 0.44; 95% CI, -0.78 to -0.11). The responsiveness of muscle stiffness was high for the affected extensor digitorum (-0.83) and moderate for the affected flexor carpi radialis (-0.71) and ulnaris (-0.77).

The responsiveness of the Myoton-3 is an important outcome measure and may serve as the foundation for therapy guidance and evaluation. The responsiveness to change of myotonometric measurements can be calculated through numeric data, provide a basis for estimates of whether the changes of muscle parameters over time are in the desired direction, and thus permit rehabilitation therapies to be adjusted accordingly. Our SRM calculations showed the affected extensor digitorum appears to be more responsive than the affected flexor carpi radialis and ulnaris in muscle tone, elasticity, and stiffness, and especially elasticity (-0.75 vs -0.44 vs -0.31). This result may arise from an emphasis on activation of wrist and finger extensor muscles elicited by the rehabilitation program the patients received. Thus, the extensor digitorum was much facilitated after treatments, and the flexor carpi muscles were not as sensitive as the extensor digitorum. Given that the ability to sustain finger extension is necessary in most functional hand activities; active finger extension is an important prognostic determinant and an early valid indicator of favorable UE function after stroke (Fritz et al., 2005; Nijland et al., 2010). Stroke patients with early finger extension after onset had a 98% probability of regaining some dexterity and a 60% probability of achieving full functional recovery of the hemiplegic arm at 6 months after stroke (Nijland et al., 2010).

4.6.5 Future directions

- Different treatment effects across treatment groups could adversely affect variability. Future studies with a larger sample size may analyze changes after specific treatment.

- Resting muscle tone during the relaxed condition does not fully quantify spasticity, which is characterized by a velocity-dependent and should be adequately performed under a dynamic state. Further studies may compare biomechanical properties of the resting muscles with the contracted muscle.
- With a sufficient sample size, a comparison of change in the myotonometric measures between patients who improved and those who did not should be analyzed separately.
- Further substantiation and generalization of these findings in larger and more diverse samples are warranted to determine clinical value of the Myoton-3.

5. Conclusion

The Myoton-3 myometer measures mechanical properties of the skeletal muscle, which may provide new insights into muscle functions to diagnose and treat muscle pathophysiology. In clinical practice and research settings, performance documented by the Myoton-3 myometer might be a useful indicator of muscle changes. This overview showed that the Myoton-3 myometer could be applied as a reliable, valid, and responsive device for objectively quantifying muscle tone, elasticity, and stiffness of resting forearm muscles in patients with stroke. These findings support the use of myotonometric measurement in stroke rehabilitation and further clinical trials.

6. Acknowledgements

This project was supported in part by the National Science Council (NSC 97-2314-B-002-008-MY3 and NSC 99-2314-B-182-014-MY3), and the National Health Research Institutes (NHRI-EX100-10010PI and NHRI-EX100-9920PI) in Taiwan.

7. References

Aarrestad, D. D., Williams, M. D., Fehrer, S. C., Mikhailenok, E., & Leonard, C. T. (2004). Intra- and interrater reliabilities of the Myotonometer when assessing the spastic condition of children with cerebral palsy. *Journal of Child Neurology,* Vol.19, No.11, (Nov 2004), pp.894-901, ISSN 0883-0738

Alhusaini, A. A., Crosbie, J., Shepherd, R. B., Dean, C. M., & Scheinberg, A. (2010). Mechanical properties of the plantarflexor musculotendinous unit during passive dorsiflexion in children with cerebral palsy compared with typically developing children. *Developmental Medicine and Child Neurology,* Vol.52, No.6, (Jun 2010), pp.e101-106, ISSN 1469-8749 (Electronic) 0012-1622 (Linking)

Ashworth, B. (1964). Preliminary trial of carisoprodol in multiple sclerosis. *The Practitioner,* Vol.192, (Apr 1964), pp.540-542, ISSN 0032-6518

Bizzini, M., & Mannion, A. F. (2003). Reliability of a new, hand-held device for assessing skeletal muscle stiffness. *Clinical Biomechanics* Vol.18, No.5, (Jun 2003), pp.459-461, ISSN 0268-0033

Bohannon, R. W., & Smith, M. B. (1987). Interrater reliability of a modified Ashworth scale of muscle spasticity. *Physical Therapy,* Vol.67, No.2, (Feb 1987), pp.206-207, ISSN 0031-9023

Brunnstrom, S. (1970). *Movement Therapy in Hemiplegia.* Harper & Row, ISBN 0-397-54808-7, New York

Chuang, L. L., Wu, C. Y., & Lin, K. C. (2012). Reliability, validity, and responsiveness of myotonometric measurement of muscle tone, elasticity, and stiffness in patients with stroke. *Archives of Physical Medicine and Rehabilitation*, Vol.93, No.3, (Mar 2012), pp.532-540, ISSN 0003-9993

Cohen, J. (1988). *Statistical power analysis for the behavioral sciences* (2nd ed.). Lawrence Erlbaum Associates, ISBN 0-8058-0283-5, Hillsdale, NJ

de Vlugt, E., de Groot, J. H., Schenkeveld, K. E., Arendzen, J. H., van der Helm, F. C., & Meskers, C. G. (2010). The relation between neuromechanical parameters and Ashworth score in stroke patients. *Journal of Neuroengineering and Rehabilitation,* Vol.7, (Jul 2010), pp.35, ISSN 1743-0003

Dietz, V., Quintern, J., & Berger, W. (1981). Electrophysiological studies of gait in spasticity and rigidity. Evidence that altered mechanical properties of muscle contribute to hypertonia. *Brain,* Vol.104, No.3, (Sep 1981), pp.431-449, ISSN 0006-8950

Ditroilo, M., Hunter, A. M., Haslam, S., & De Vito, G. (2011). The effectiveness of two novel techniques in establishing the mechanical and contractile responses of biceps femoris. *Physiological Measurement,* Vol.32, No.8, (Aug 2011), pp.1315-1326, ISSN 1361-6579 (Electronic) 0967-3334 (Linking)

Fess, E. E., & Moran, C. A. (1981). *Clinical assessment recommendations.* American Society of Hand Therapists, Indianapolis.

Folstein, M. F., Folstein, S. E., & McHugh, P. R. (1975). "Mini-mental state". A practical method for grading the cognitive state of patients for the clinician. *Journal of Psychiatric Research,* Vol.12, No.3, (Nov 1975), pp.189-198, ISSN 0022-3956

Fritz, S. L., Light, K. E., Patterson, T. S., Behrman, A. L., & Davis, S. B. (2005). Active finger extension predicts outcomes after constraint-induced movement therapy for individuals with hemiparesis after stroke. *Stroke,* Vol.36, No.6, (Jun 2005), pp.1172-1177, ISSN 1524-4628 (Electronic) 0039-2499 (Linking)

Gapeyeva, H., & Vain, A. (2008). *Methodical guide: Principles of applying Myoton in physical medicine and rehabilitation.* Muomeetria Ltd, Tartu, Estonia

Gavronski, G., Veraksits, A., Vasar, E., & Maaroos, J. (2007). Evaluation of viscoelastic parameters of the skeletal muscles in junior triathletes. *Physiological Measurement,* Vol.28, No.6, (Jun 2007), pp.625-637, ISSN 0967-3334

Gregson, J. M., Leathley, M. J., Moore, A. P., Smith, T. L., Sharma, A. K., & Watkins, C. L. (2000). Reliability of measurements of muscle tone and muscle power in stroke patients. *Age and Ageing,* Vol.29, No.3, (May 2000), pp.223-228, ISSN 0002-0729

Gubler-Hanna, C., Laskin, J., Marx, B. J., & Leonard, C. T. (2007). Construct validity of myotonometric measurements of muscle compliance as a measure of strength. *Physiological Measurement,* Vol.28, No.8, (Aug 2007), pp.913-924, ISSN 0967-3334

Haas, B. M., & Crow, J. L. (1995). Towards a clinical measurement of spasticity? *Physiotherapy,* Vol.81, No.8, (Aug 1995), pp.474-479, ISSN 0031-9406

Hafer-Macko, C. E., Ryan, A. S., Ivey, F. M., & Macko, R. F. (2008). Skeletal muscle changes after hemiparetic stroke and potential beneficial effects of exercise intervention strategies. *Journal of Rehabilitation Research & Development,* Vol.45, No.2 (Feb 2008), pp.261-272, ISSN 1938-1352 (Electronic) 0748-7711 (Linking)

Haidar, S. G., Kumar, D., Bassi, R. S., & Deshmukh, S. C. (2004). Average versus maximum grip strength: which is more consistent? *The Journal of Hand Surgery,* Vol.29, No.1, (Feb 2004), pp.82-84, ISSN 0266-7681

Hoang, P. D., Herbert, R. D., & Gandevia, S. C. (2007). Effects of eccentric exercise on passive mechanical properties of human gastrocnemius in vivo. *Medicine and Science in Sports and Exercise,* Vol.39, No.5, (May 2007), pp.849-857, ISSN 0195-9131

Hsieh, Y. W., Wu, C. Y., Lin, K. C., Chang, Y. F., Chen, C. L., & Liu, J. S. (2009). Responsiveness and validity of three outcome measures of motor function after stroke rehabilitation. *Stroke,* Vol.40, No.4, (Apr 2009), pp.1386-1391, ISSN 1524-4628

Huang, S. Y., Di Santo, M., Wadden, K. P., Cappa, D. F., Alkanani, T., & Behm, D. G. (2010). Short-duration massage at the hamstrings musculotendinous junction induces greater range of motion. *Journal of Strength and Conditioning Research,* Vol.24, No.7, (Jul 2010), pp.1917-1924, ISSN 1533-4287 (Electronic) 1064-8011 (Linking).

Ianieri, G., Saggini, R., Marvulli, R., Tondi, G., Aprile, A., Ranieri, M., Benedetto, G., Altini, S., Lancioni, G. E., Goffredo, L., Bellomo, R. G., Megna, M., & Megna, G. (2009). New approach in the assessment of the tone, elasticity and the muscular resistance: nominal scales vs MYOTON. *International Journal of Immunopathology and Pharmacology,* Vol.22, No.3 Suppl, (Jul-Sep 2009), pp.21-24, ISSN 0394-6320

Katz, R. T., & Rymer, W. Z. (1989). Spastic hypertonia: mechanisms and measurement. *Archives of Physical Medicine and Rehabilitation,* Vol.70, No.2, (Feb 1989), pp.144-155, ISSN 0003-9993

Lance, J. W. (1980). *Spasticity: Disordered motor control.* Year Book Publishers, Chicago, IL.

Lee, K. C., Carson, L., Kinnin, E., & Patterson, V. (1989). The Ashworth Scale: A reliable and reproducible method of measuring spasticity. *Neurorehabilitation and Neural Repair,* Vol.3, No.4, (Dec 1989), pp.205-209.

Leonard, C. T., Brown, J. S., Price, T. R., Queen, S. A., & Mikhailenok, E. L. (2004). Comparison of surface electromyography and myotonometric measurements during voluntary isometric contractions. *Journal of Electromyography and Kinesiology,* Vol.14, No.6, (Dec 2004), pp.709-714, ISSN 1050-6411

Leonard, C. T., Deshner, W. P., Romo, J. W., Suoja, E. S., Fehrer, S. C., & Mikhailenok, E. L. (2003). Myotonometer intra- and interrater reliabilities. *Archives of Physical Medicine and Rehabilitation,* Vol.84, No.6, (Jun 2003), pp.928-932, ISSN 0003-9993

Leonard, C. T., Stephens, J. U., & Stroppel, S. L. (2001). Assessing the spastic condition of individuals with upper motoneuron involvement: validity of the myotonometer. *Archives of Physical Medicine and Rehabilitation,* Vol.82, No.10, (Oct 2001), pp.1416-1420, ISSN 0003-9993

Lidstrom, A., Ahlsten, G., Hirchfeld, H., & Norrlin, S. (2009). Intrarater and interrater reliability of Myotonometer measurements of muscle tone in children. *Journal of Child Neurology,* Vol.24, No.3, (Mar 2009), pp.267-274, ISSN 1708-8283 (Electronic) 0883-0738 (Linking)

Lin, K. C., Chuang, L. L., Wu, C. Y., Hsieh, Y. W., & Chang, W. Y. (2010). Responsiveness and validity of three dexterous function measures in stroke rehabilitation. *Journal of Rehabilitation Research & Development,* Vol.47, No.6, (Sep 2010), pp.563-571, ISSN 1938-1352 (Electronic) 0748-7711 (Linking).

Lyle, R. C. (1981). A performance test for assessment of upper limb function in physical rehabilitation treatment and research. *International Journal of Rehabilitation Research,* Vol.4, No.4, (Dec 1981), pp.483-492.

Magnusson, S. P. (1998). Passive properties of human skeletal muscle during stretch maneuvers. A review. *Scandinavian Journal of Medicine & Science in Sports*, Vol.8, No.2, (Apr 1998), pp.65-77, ISSN 0905-7188

Marusiak, J., Kisiel-Sajewicz, K., Jaskolska, A., & Jaskolski, A. (2010). Higher muscle passive stiffness in Parkinson's disease patients than in controls measured by myotonometry. *Archives of Physical Medicine and Rehabilitation*, Vol.91, No.5, (May 2010), pp.800-802, ISSN 1532-821X (Electronic) 0003-9993 (Linking)

Masi, A. T., & Hannon, J. C. (2008). Human resting muscle tone (HRMT): narrative introduction and modern concepts. *Journal of Bodywork and Movement Therapies*, Vol.12, No.4, (Oct 2008), pp.320-332, ISSN 1532-9283 (Electronic) 1360-8592 (Linking)

Mathiowetz, V., Kashman, N., Volland, G., Weber, K., Dowe, M., & Rogers, S. (1985). Grip and pinch strength: normative data for adults. *Archives of Physical Medicine and Rehabilitation*, Vol.66, No.2, (Feb 1985), pp.69-74, ISSN 0003-9993

Mathiowetz, V., Weber, K., Volland, G., & Kashman, N. (1984). Reliability and validity of grip and pinch strength evaluations. *The Journal of Hand Surgery*, Vol.9, No.2, (Mar 1984), pp.222-226, ISSN 0363-5023

Nijland, R. H., van Wegen, E. E., Harmeling-van der Wel, B. C., & Kwakkel, G. (2010). Presence of finger extension and shoulder abduction within 72 hours after stroke predicts functional recovery: early prediction of functional outcome after stroke: the EPOS cohort study. *Stroke*, Vol.41, No.4, (Apr 2010), pp.745-750, ISSN 1524-4628 (Electronic) 0039-2499 (Linking)

Nordez, A., Gennisson, J. L., Casari, P., Catheline, S., & Cornu, C. (2008). Characterization of muscle belly elastic properties during passive stretching using transient elastography. *Journal of Biomechanics*, Vol.41, No.10, (Jul 2008), pp.2305-2311, ISSN 0021-9290

O'Dwyer, N. J., Ada, L., & Neilson, P. D. (1996). Spasticity and muscle contracture following stroke. *Brain*, Vol, 119, No.5, pp.1737-1749, ISSN 1460-2156

Pandyan, A. D., Johnson, G. R., Price, C. I., Curless, R. H., Barnes, M. P., & Rodgers, H. (1999). A review of the properties and limitations of the Ashworth and modified Ashworth Scales as measures of spasticity. *Clinical Rehabilitation*, Vol.13, No.5, (Oct 1999), pp.373-383, ISSN 0269-2155

Panjabi, M. M. (1992). The stabilizing system of the spine. Part I. Function, dysfunction, adaptation, and enhancement. *Journal of Spinal Disorders*, Vol.5, No.4, (Dec 1992), pp.383-389; discussion 397, ISSN 0895-0385

Platz, T., Pinkowski, C., van Wijck, F., Kim, I. H., di Bella, P., & Johnson, G. (2005). Reliability and validity of arm function assessment with standardized guidelines for the Fugl-Meyer Test, Action Research Arm Test and Box and Block Test: a multicentre study. *Clinical Rehabilitation*, Vol.19, No.4, (Jun 2005), pp.404-411, ISSN 1477-0873

Pomeroy, V. M., Dean, D., Sykes, L., Faragher, E. B., Yates, M., Tyrrell, P. J., Moss, S., & Tallis, R. C. (2000). The unreliability of clinical measures of muscle tone: implications for stroke therapy. *Age and Ageing*, Vol.29, No.3, (May 2000), pp.229-233.

Portney, L. G., & Watkins, M. P. (2009). *Foundations of clinical research: Applications to practice* (3rd ed.). Pearson/Prentice Hall, Upper Saddle River, ISBN 0131716409, NJ.

Pynsent, P. B. (2001). Choosing an outcome measure. *The Journal of Bone and Joint Surgery. British Volume,* Vol.83, No.6, (Aug 2001), pp.792-794, ISSN 0301-620X (Print).

Rabadi, M. H., & Rabadi, F. M. (2006). Comparison of the Action Research Arm Test and the Fugl-Meyer Assessment as measures of upper-extremity motor weakness after stroke. *Archives of Physical Medicine and Rehabilitation,* Vol.87, No.7, (Jul 2006), pp.962-966.

Ratsep, T., & Asser, T. (2011). Changes in viscoelastic properties of skeletal muscles induced by subthalamic stimulation in patients with Parkinson's disease. *Clinical Biomechanics (Bristol, Avon),* Vol.26, No.2, (Feb 2011), pp.213-217, ISSN 1879-1271 (Electronic) 0268-0033 (Linking)

Reisman, S., Allen, T. J., & Proske, U. (2009). Changes in passive tension after stretch of unexercised and eccentrically exercised human plantarflexor muscles. *Experimental Brain Research,* Vol.193, No.4, (Mar 2009), pp.545-554, ISSN 1432-1106 (Electronic) 0014-4819 (Linking).

Roja, Z., Kalkis, V., Vain, A., Kalkis, H., & Eglite, M. (2006). Assessment of skeletal muscle fatigue of road maintenance workers based on heart rate monitoring and myotonometry. *Journal of Occupational Medicine and Toxicology,* Vol.1, (July 2006), pp.20, ISSN 1745-6673 (Electronic)

Rydahl, S. J., & Brouwer, B. J. (2004). Ankle stiffness and tissue compliance in stroke survivors: a validation of myotonometer measurements. *Archives of Physical Medicine and Rehabilitation,* Vol.85, No.10, (Oct 2004), pp.1631-1637, ISSN 0003-9993

Shaw, L. C., Price, C. I., van Wijck, F. M., Shackley, P., Steen, N., Barnes, M. P., Ford, G. A., Graham, L. A., & Rodgers, H. (2011). Botulinum Toxin for the Upper Limb after Stroke (BoTULS) Trial: effect on impairment, activity limitation, and pain. *Stroke,* Vol.42, No.5, (May 2011), pp.1371-1379, ISSN 1524-4628 (Electronic) 0039-2499 (Linking)

Sheean, G., & McGuire, J. R. (2009). Spastic hypertonia and movement disorders: Pathophysiology, clinical presentation, and quantification. *PM & R: The Journal of Injury, Function, and Rehabilitation,* Vol.1, No.9 (Sep 2009), pp.827-833, ISSN 1934-1482

Simons, D. G., & Mense, S. (1998). Understanding and measurement of muscle tone as related to clinical muscle pain. *Pain,* Vol.75, No.1, (Mar 1998), pp.1-17, ISSN 0304-3959

Sjostrom, M., Fugl-Meyer, A. R., Nordin, G., & Wahlby, L. (1980). Post-stroke hemiplegia; crural muscle strength and structure. *Scandinavian Journal of Rehabilitation Medicine. Supplement,* Vol.7, (Jul 1980), pp.53-67, ISSN 0346-8720

Sommerfeld, D. K., Eek, E. U.-B., Svensson, A.-K., Holmqvist, L. W., & von Arbin, M. H. (2004). Spasticity after stroke: its occurrence and association with motor impairments and activity limitations. *Stroke,* Vol.35, No.1, (Jan 2004), pp.134-139, ISSN 0039-2499

Svantesson, U., Takahashi, H., Carlsson, U., Danielsson, A., & Sunnerhagen, K. S. (2000). Muscle and tendon stiffness in patients with upper motor neuron lesion following a stroke. *European Journal of Applied Physiology,* Vol.82, No.4, (Jul 2000), pp.275-279, ISSN 1439-6319

Vain, A. (1995). Estimation of the functional state of skeletal muscle. In P. H. Veltink & H.B.K. Boom, (Eds.), *Control of ambulation using functional neuromuscular stimulation.* (pp. 51-55). University of Twente Press, ISBN 9036507340, 9789036507349, Enschede, Netherlands

van der Lee, J. H., Beckerman, H., Lankhorst, G. J., & Bouter, L. M. (2001). The responsiveness of the Action Research Arm test and the Fugl-Meyer Assessment scale in chronic stroke patients. *Journal of Rehabilitation Medicine,* Vol.33, No.3, (Mar 2001), pp.110-113, ISSN 1650-1977

Viir, R., Laiho, K., Kramarenko, J., & Mikkelson, M. (2006). Repeatability of trapezius muscle tone assessment by a myometric method. *Journal of Mechanics in Medicine and Biology,* Vol.6, No.2, (Feb 2006), pp.215-228, ISSN 0219-5194

Wade, D. T. (1992). *Measurement in neurological rehabilitation.* Oxford: Oxford Medical Publications, ISBN 978-0-323-04621-3, New York.

Ward, A. B. (2000). Assessment of muscle tone. *Age and Ageing,* Vol.29, No.5, (Sep 2000), pp.385-386, ISSN 0002-0729

Weir, J. P. (2005). Quantifying test-retest reliability using the intraclass correlation coefficient and the SEM. *Journal of Strength and Conditioning Research,* Vol.19, No.1, (Feb 2005), pp.231-240, ISSN 1064-8011

Whitehead, N. P., Weerakkody, N. S., Gregory, J. E., Morgan, D. L., & Proske, U. (2001). Changes in passive tension of muscle in humans and animals after eccentric exercise. *Journal of Physiology,* Vol.533, No.Pt 2, (Jun 2001), pp.593-604, ISSN 0022-3751

4

Validity and Reliability of a Hand-Held Dynamometer for Dynamic Muscle Strength Assessment

Lan Le-Ngoc[1] and Jessica Janssen[2]
[1]*Industrial Research Ltd, Christchurch*
[2]*Burwood Academy of Independent Living, Christchurch*
New Zealand

1. Introduction

An important component of physical therapy is to conduct assessment of a patient's mobility including muscle strength and joint range of motion (ROM).

The purposes of this study were to investigate the possibility of measuring dynamic muscle strength using a new hand-held device and to assess its validity and reliability. If proven valid and reliable, this device will provide a practical tool for physical therapists to perform dynamic muscle assessment in a clinical setting.

The current standard clinical evaluation and diagnostic tool for muscle strength assessment is the manual muscle testing (MMT) method, using a 5-point grading scale (Clarkson (2000); Petty (2011)). Although it has been a clinically useful tool for over forty years, its accuracy and reliability remains questionable (Cuthbert & Goodheart (2007); Frese et al. (1987)).

To overcome the limitations of the MMT, isometric hand-held dynamometers (HHD) have been developed to aid therapists in clinics (Andrews (1991)). HHDs are generally small and portable, and measure strength objectively in kilograms, pounds or newtons. The clinician holds the HHD between his or her force-applying hand and the patient's limb segment. The clinician stabilises the limb segment while encouraging the patient to exert as much force against the device as possible and the maximum force is recorded by the HHD. Such devices have been proven to have good to excellent reliability in different populations (Andrews (1991); Bohannon & Andrews (1987); Stark et al. (2011)). In a single test, however, they can assess the strength of a patient at only one joint angle, rather than through the patient's entire ROM. Although this technique provides a crucial tool for clinical quantification of joint strength at a fixed static position (isometric), it cannot measure properties from dynamic muscle performance assessments.

Isokinetic dynamometers, such as the Cybex (USA) or the Biodex (USA), are considered as the gold standard in simultaneous strength and angle measurements for the evaluation of dynamic muscular performance (Kannus (1994); Baltzopoulos & Brodie (1989); Osternig (1986); Lund et al. (2005); Drouin et al. (2004)). Strength profiles showing instantaneous torque versus joint angle are generated and a number of properties such as dynamic peak torque, peak torque angle, angle-specific torque, power, and energy used can be determined. The dynamic strength profiles can also be used to detect weaknesses over small regions of a specific joint's ROM. Other advantages of the isokinetic dynamometer over the current isometric HHDs are that assessor's strength is not an issue; the subject is stabilized consistently during testing; and the joint angle and strength are measured simultaneously during testing (Lund et al. (2005); Martin et al. (2006); Harlaar et al. (1996)). Disadvantages of these devices are their size and cost, which make them impractical for routine clinical examinations (Li et al. (2006);Mital et al. (1995)).

Recognising the needs for better clinical strength assessment tools, there have been a number of attempts to incorporate angle measurement in the strength assessment (Li et al. (2006); Roebroeck et al. (1998)). However, there have been no published results on the use of a single hand-held device to perform dynamic strength measurements on human subjects. A new device, referred to as the IRL-HHD (Fig. 1), is a single hand-held device that can measure force and angle simultaneously while the joint moves through its ROM[1]. The ability to measure force and angle simultaneously means that it can measure energy or power in a similar manner to an isokinetic dynamometer. In order for the IRL-HHD to capture dynamic joint strength, the assessor must provide sufficient force to resist the limb movement, but also allow the limb to move at a constant and controllable pace. This is not a trivial task and the assessor may not be able to concentrate on keeping the device in perfect alignment with the limb. The algorithm used in the IRL-HHD can measure the required joint angle accurately without having to maintain the alignment of the longitudinal axis of the device with respect to the limb. In some cases, this feature allows the joint to reach its full ROM (see Fig. 2 for an example of measuring concentric elbow flexion where the longitudinal axis of the IRL-HHD does not have to be aligned with the forearm). The IRL-HHD and the assessment techniques have been shown to be reliable and valid by measuring concentric flexion of a simulated mechanical arm, which was used to eliminate the effects of human variability (Janssen & Le-Ngoc (2009)).

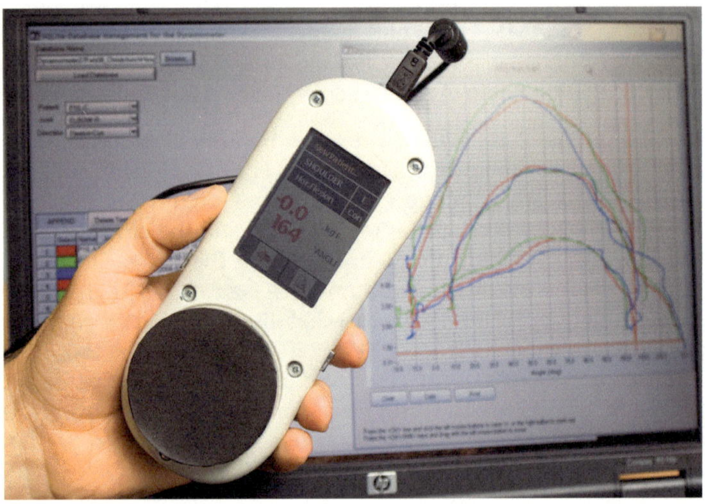

Fig. 1. IRL Hand-held dynamometer.

This article describes the validity and reliability trials of the device to measure concentric elbow flexion and concentric knee extension on human subjects. Other possible uses of the IRL-HHD in clinical and on-field assessments are also discussed.

[1] Patent WO/2011/002315 - Inventor: Industrial Research Ltd (IRL)

2. Validity and reliability of dynamic muscle strength assessment

This section describes the test protocol and the results of using the IRL-HHD to perform concentric elbow flexion and concentric knee extension assessment on human subjects.

2.1 Instrumentation

Two dynamometers, the IRL-HHD and the isokinetic dynamometer (Biodex), were used to measure maximal concentric strength for elbow flexion and knee extension. The Biodex measurements were corrected for the effect of gravity caused by the Biodex lever arm. For the IRL-HHD tests, a seat and an arm rest attached to a plinth were used to position and restrain the participants in a similar manner to the tests carried out using the Biodex (see Fig. 2 and Fig. 3).

2.2 Protocol

A registered physiotherapist conducted the tests using the IRL-HHD and another registered physiotherapist performed the Biodex tests. Both therapists were blinded from the outcome measures.

2.2.1 Participants

Fifteen able-bodied, healthy adults participated in this study, which was approved by the University of Otago (New Zealand) Ethics Committee. All participants provided informed written consent before testing.

2.2.2 Design

There were two test sessions for each participant using the IRL-HHD, and one test session using the Biodex. Each test session comprised one sub-maximal contraction, and three repeated maximal strength contractions to perform right elbow flexion and right knee extension. Each measurement was followed by a one minute rest period. The order of sessions was randomized for each participant, and within each session the order in which joints were tested was randomized. The participants were given five minutes rest between each test session to prevent fatigue.

The distances from the centre of the force pad to the rotational axis of elbow and knee were recorded for each participant and used to convert measured forces into joint torques. Peak torque, peak torque angle and total work were obtained from the torque versus joint angle curves recorded by both dynamometers.

A three-stage procedure was followed to record strength versus joint angle data using the IRL-HDD:

- Defining the zero position of the joint;
- Moving the joint to the start position, positioning the device to resist the limb motion and commencing the measurement;
- Instructing the participant to exert maximal muscular contraction while providing a resistance to control the movement of the joint, and stopping the measurement when the participant reaches the end of joint movement.

For concentric elbow flexion, the participant was seated beside the end of the plinth, and the right arm was strapped to an arm rest at 60° shoulder flexion and 30° shoulder abduction

(Fig. 2). The zero position of the elbow was identified by placing the device lengthwise on a reference line between the acromion and the lateral epicondyle of the humerus. The device was placed with the force pad 2 cm proximal of the wrist while the arm was fully extended. It is possible to have a negative start angle, which is a measure of elbow hyperextension.

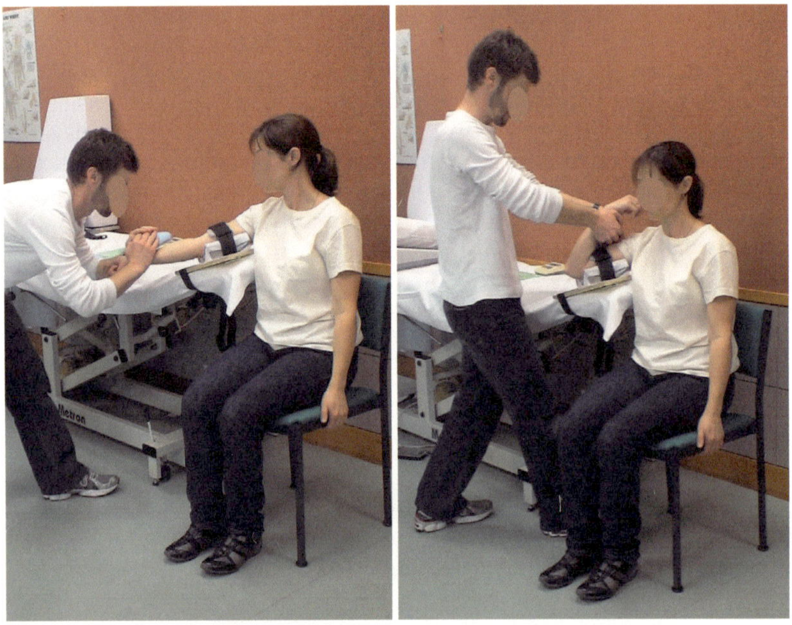

(a) Start and end position of the IRL-HHD measurement

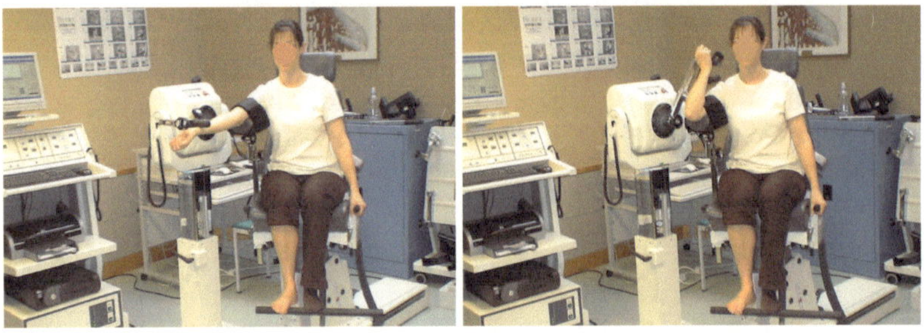

(b) Start and end position of the Biodex measurement

Fig. 2. Concentric elbow flexion measurements with the IRL-HHD and the Biodex.

For concentric knee extension, the participant was seated using the same arrangement as on the Biodex (Fig. 3). The zero position was set against a horizontal surface. The device was placed with the force pad 10 cm proximal of the medial malleolus and the leg was moved to the starting position (110° knee flexion) before commencing the measurement.

The isokinetic mode of the Biodex was used for testing with a maximum speed of 60°/s. In this mode, the start and end ROM had to be set before starting the test. For elbow flexion, the zero elbow position was set so that the participant's arm was supported at 60° shoulder flexion and 30° shoulder abduction (Fig. 2). Unfortunately, the Biodex strap restricted some participants from reaching end ROM, so it was not possible to provide a comparison of elbow

ROM measurements between the IRL-HHD and the Biodex. For knee extension, the Biodex chair and the fixture beneath the chair prevented participants from reaching full knee flexion. In order to provide a meaningful comparison of the peak torque angle, the starting position of the knee extension was set at the maximum possible knee flexion angle but not greater than 110°. Because of this preset starting position, it was not meaningful to report knee ROM measurements using the Biodex.

During testing, the physiotherapist manually recorded any unusual events, such as loss of control, or excessive movement of the IRL-HHD. These tests were discarded from the data set, which was justified on the basis that it would be standard clinical practice to ignore erroneous tests at the time of testing.

The ability of the therapist to maintain the control of the dynamic measurement is discussed in Section 4.1.

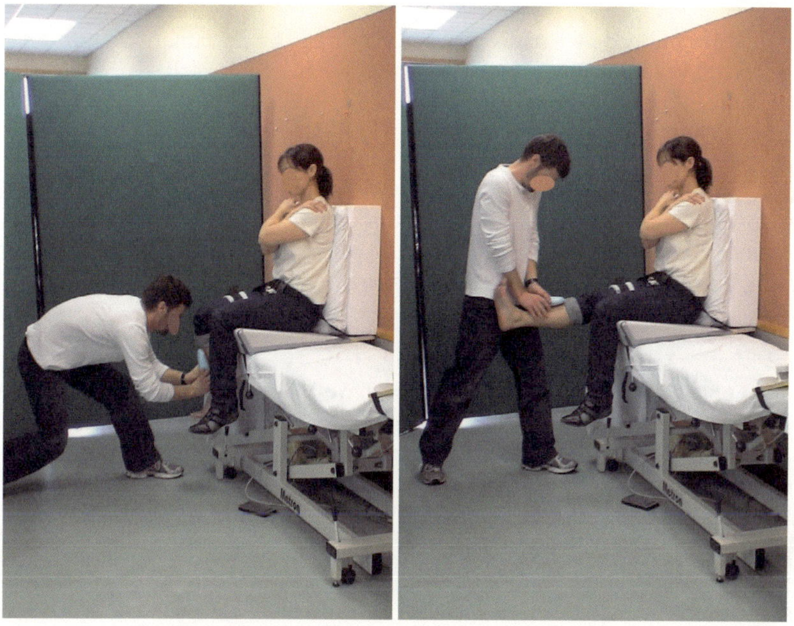

(a) Start and end position of the IRL-HHD measurement

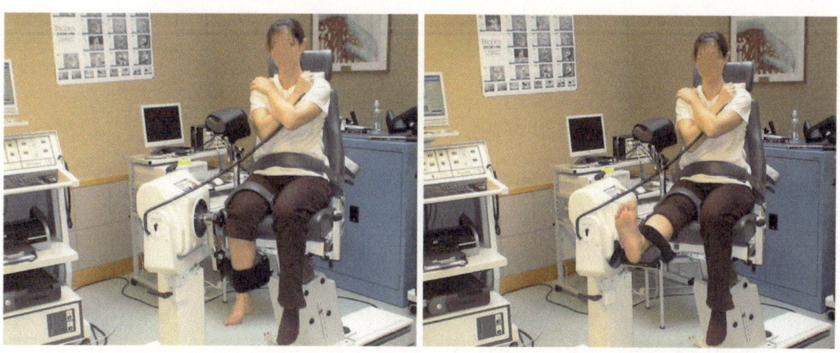

(b) Start and end position of the Biodex measurement

Fig. 3. Concentric knee extension measurements with the IRL-HHD and the Biodex.

2.3 Statistical analysis

2.3.1 Descriptive statistics

Descriptive statistics of muscle torques, joint angles and muscular work are presented in Nm, degrees (°) and J respectively. Torque is calculated from the measured peak force times the length from the centre of the force pad to the rotational axis of the elbow or knee. Work is defined as output of mechanical energy, that is, externally applied force multiplied by the distance through which it is applied. In the concentric measurements, work can be found by calculating the area under the torque versus angular displacement curve. Mean and standard deviations (SDs) are reported. All analyses were performed using the Matlab software package (USA).

2.3.2 Intratester reliability

The degree of correlation between six repetitions of all the maximal strength tests using the IRL-HHD is calculated with the intraclass correlation co-efficient ($ICC_{1,1}$) defined by Schrout and Fleiss (1979). The same test was performed on the three repetitions of the Biodex. The most critical reliability assessment is the $ICC_{1,1}$, which assumes that every individual measurement is independent and the error of measurement is assumed to be normally distributed. Other authors have used $ICC_{2,1}$ for their reliability measurement, which tends to give more optimistic values than $ICC_{1,1}$. In this article all $ICC_{1,1}$ results are almost equal to the $ICC_{2,1}$ values. According to Fleiss (1986), the reliability of an ICC over 0.75 is considered to be excellent, and between 0.4-0.75 as fair to good.

2.3.3 Validity

The agreement between the two devices can be quantified using the Bland-Altman 95% limits of agreement (LOA) method (Bland & Altman (1986)). The LOA method is based on the mean and SD of the differences between the measurements by the two devices. For repeated measurements, a one-way ANOVA is performed for each device separately. Outcomes of the one-way ANOVA are then used to calculate the lower and upper LOA (mean $\pm$ 1.96 times SD)(Bland & Altman (2007)).

3. Results

3.1 Descriptive Statistics

Five men and ten women participated in this research. The participants' ages ranged from 23 to 45 years (mean$\pm$SD, 32.6$\pm$7.2y). Fig. 4 shows typical strength profile plots between the IRL-HHD and the Biodex for one participant. Although the shape of torque versus angle graphs were not the same for the IRL-HHD and the Biodex, both methods show consistency in repeated measurements.

Fig. 5 shows the speed of all measurements obtained with the IRL-HHD. It shows that the physiotherapist was able to control the speed of each measurement very well for the elbow flexion. Only two participants generated speeds more than 100°/s while nine generated speeds less than 80°/s. It was more difficult for the physiotherapist to control the speed for the knee extension and five participants generated speed greater than 100°/s. The range of speeds for those participants was also greater, suggesting that the physiotherapist was not in control of all the tests. Since the speed is controlled entirely from the perception of the assessor, an error of $\pm$20°/s is considered to be reasonable in this study.

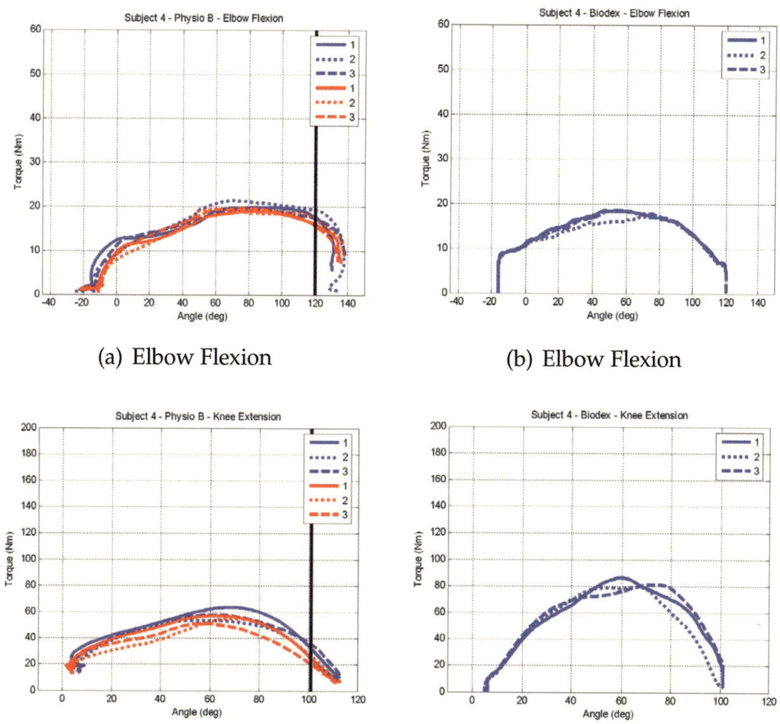

(a) Elbow Flexion

(b) Elbow Flexion

(c) Knee Extension

(d) Knee Extension

Fig. 4. Strength profiles of one participant for concentric elbow flexion and knee extension obtained from the IRL-HHD (a, c) and the Biodex (b, d).

Fig. 6 shows scatter graphs of the mean peak torque and mean work between the Biodex (x-axis) and the IRL-HHD (y-axis) for elbow flexion, and Fig. 7 shows the corresponding data for knee extension. The error bars show the individual SDs for the Biodex and the IRL-HHD. It is interesting to note that the error bars for the Biodex are generally larger than those for the IRL-HHD, indicating that variability of the tested participants is a significant factor in strength measurements. For elbow flexion, fourteen out of fifteen participants generated peak torques less than 50 Nm. For knee extension, the physiotherapist was unable to resist any torque greater than 100 Nm, whereas five participants generated more than 100 Nm on the Biodex.

3.2 Intratester reliability

Six repeated measurements with the IRL-HHD and three with the Biodex were used to calculate the ICCs and their 95% confidence intervals. The results are shown in Table 1. The $ICC_{1,1}$ values of both devices indicates excellent intratester reliability in the peak torque and work for both elbow flexion and knee extension. Repeatability of the peak torque angle of both tests by both devices is rated fair to good. However the confidence intervals indicates that only the knee peak torque angle obtained from the Biodex can be considered as fair to good, while all other peak torque angle measurements are poor. To determine if the mean of three measurements is a more reliable measure of the peak torque angle, the $ICCs_{1,3}$ of

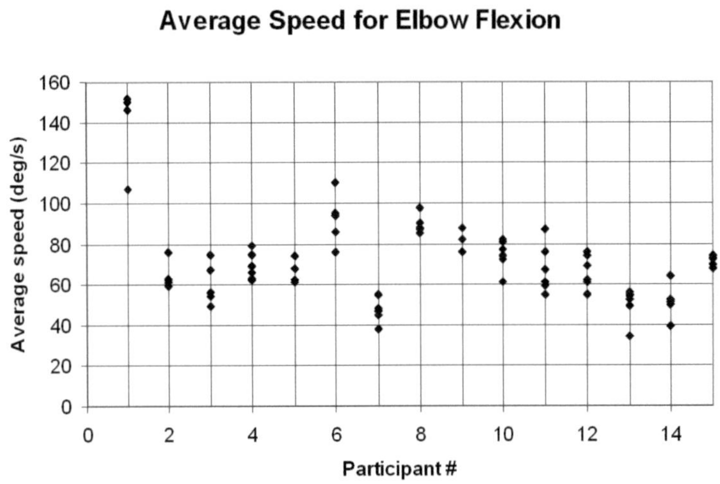

(a) Elbow Flexion

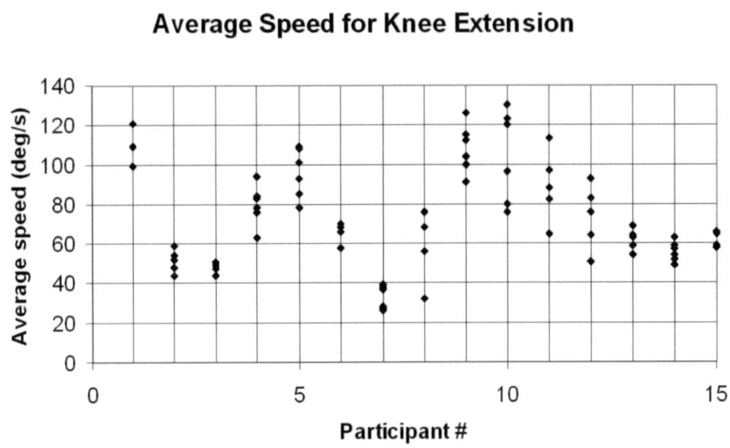

(b) Knee Extension

Fig. 5. Average speeds obtained with the IRL-HHD.

the peak torque angles in the first session of the IRL-HHD tests were found to be 0.80 (0.50, 0.93) for elbow flexion and 0.75 (0.38, 0.91) for knee extension which are within the range of excellent.

3.3 Validity

The overall mean differences and their SDs between the two devices, and all lower and upper LOA values are shown in Table 2. The differences were calculated by subtracting the Biodex values from the corresponding IRL-HHD values, hence a negative value indicates that the IRL-HHD measurement is smaller than the Biodex measurement. The table also shows the LOA for screened data as will be discussed in Section 4.3.

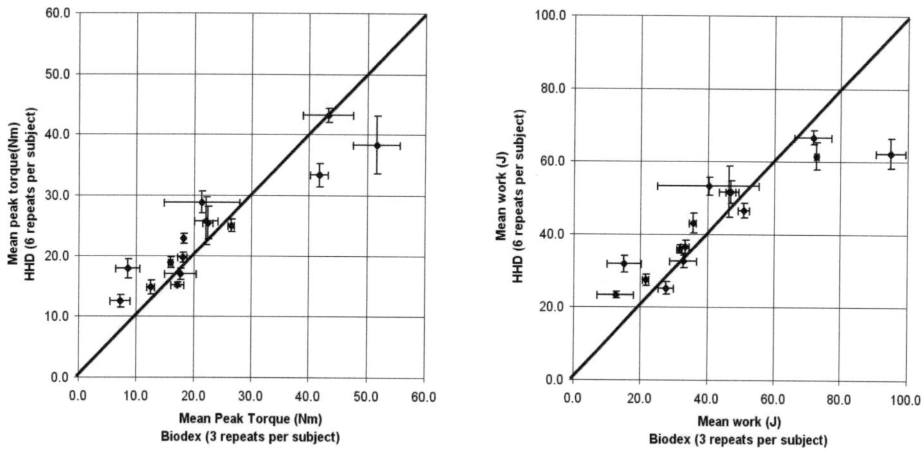

(a) Mean peak torque (b) Mean work

Fig. 6. Scatter plots of (a) mean peak torque and (b) mean work for elbow flexion as measured by Biodex and IRL-HHD. The solid lines are the equality lines.

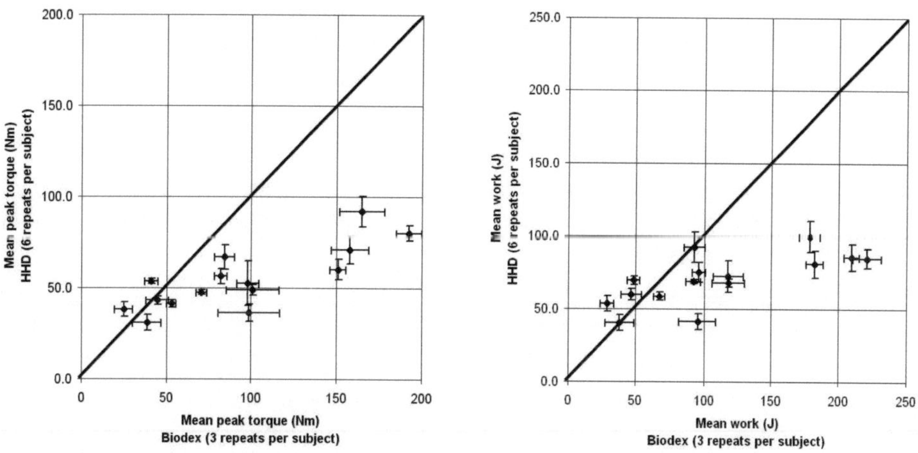

(a) Mean peak torque (b) Mean work

Fig. 7. Scatter plots of (a) mean peak torque and (b) mean work for knee extension as measured by Biodex and IRL-HHD. The solid lines are the equality lines.

4. Discussion

4.1 Descriptive statistics

The graphs of torque versus angle in Fig. 4 suggest that the standardized methods of measurement using the IRL-HHD provided reliable concentric measurement. Speed variation during a single test using the IRL-HHD may be a factor in producing different shapes of the torque-angle curves between the IRL-HHD and the Biodex.

Joint Movement	Measurements	IRL-HHD	Biodex	IRL-HHD Session 1
Elbow flexion	PT	0.95(0.91 to 0.98)	0.96(0.90 to 0.98)	
	PT Angle	0.41(0.20 to 0.68)	0.56(0.25 to 0.81)	0.80(0.50 to 0.93)
	Work	0.97(0.93 to 0.99)	0.95(0.88 to 0.98)	
Knee extension	PT	0.99(0.94 to 0.99)	0.97(0.93 to 0.99)	
	PT Angle	0.46(0.24 to 0.71)	0.67(0.41 to 0.86)	0.75(0.38 to 0.91)
	Work	0.86(0.73 to 0.94)	0.98(0.96 to 0.99)	

NOTE. 95% confidence intervals shown in parenthesis
Abbreviation: PT, peak torque.

Table 1. $ICC_{1,1}$ for six repetitions with the IRL-HHD and three repetitions with the Biodex, and $ICC_{1,3}$ for the first session with the IRL-HHD.

	Elbow flexion			Knee extension		
	PT	PT angle	Work	PT	PT angle	Work
Mean difference (SD)	1.0(6.4)	24(23)	1.0(12.8)	-39.1(40.3)	2(14)	-38.9(52.7)
95% LOA for all data	-11.6, 13.5	-21, 69	-24.1, 26.0	-118.2, 40.0	-26, 30	-142.0, 64.5
95% LOA for screened data	-7.0, 9.9	-15, 53	-12.4, 16.2	-23.1, 28.7	-16, 41	-13.1, 41.0

Table 2. Agreement between the IRL-HHD and the Biodex for assessing elbow flexion and knee extension.

An angular speed measurement greater than 100°/s indicates that the physiotherapist is overpowered by the participant and that the result is likely to be invalid. Fig. 5 shows that it is possible for a trained assessor to control the concentric assessment speed to within ±20°/s from a target speed of 60°/s, provided that the force generated by the subject is less than the strength limit of the assessor.

Further examination shows that most of the variability in the Biodex arises from the first test in a series of three repeats being sub-maximal. It is recommended for future study that the warm-up phase should consist of more than one sub-maximal concentric movement.

For knee extension, the physiotherapist was unable to resist any torque greater than 100 Nm, whereas five participants generated more than 100 Nm on the Biodex. From the elbow tests, the assessor was overpowered by one participant, who generated 52 Nm peak torque, but was able to perform tests satisfactorily at 43 Nm peak torque, suggesting that the strength limit of this assessor is between 43 Nm and 52 Nm for elbow flexion (approximately 200 N to 250 N in force). Several authors have specified minimum upper limits of assessor's strength necessary for performing isometric measurements using an HHD (Wikholm & Bohannon (1991)). A conservative value is 12 kg of resistive force (Edwards & McDonnell (1974)) while others have suggested a value of 30 kg force (Hyde et al. (1983)). van der Ploeg et al. (1984) stated that an HHD range beyond 220 N is not useful due to stabilization and strength issues. The upper limit of the assessor's strength in this study is in agreement with the published results for isometric measurements. The torque limit of this assessor is expected to be between 52 Nm and 65 Nm for knee extension. Only four of the fifteen participants (27%) generated less than 52 Nm for knee extension, hence it may be concluded that the IRL-HHD and the test protocol described in this article is not feasible for general use in measuring knee extension of healthy adults. Most participants generated peak elbow fexion torques less than 50 Nm, suggesting that the IRL-HHD can be used to measure concentric strength of upper extremities or minor muscle groups in general healthy population. It may also be possible to use the IRL-HHD to assess children's concentric strength and subjects with strength deficiency resulting from conditions such as stroke or spinal cord injury.

4.2 Intratester reliability

Intratester reliabilities of peak torque and work are excellent in both elbow and knee measurements with the IRL-HHD and with the Biodex, while the intratester reliabilities of peak torque angle are poor for the IRL-HHD. The intratester reliabilities of the peak torque angle using the Biodex are slightly better than those obtained with the IRL-HHD. The $ICCs_{1,3}$ of the first sessions using the IRL-HHD indicates a significant improvement in the reliability of measuring the peak torque angle. These values suggest that peak torque angle should be measured by taking the mean of three repeated tests. The $ICCs_{1,3}$ for peak torque angle are within the range of excellent for both elbow flexion and knee extension.

4.3 Validity

The conventional method of assessing and grading muscle strength is the manual muscle test. In this study, all of the participants would be rated with a score of 5 as they were all healthy. Quantitative assessments of concentric strength are mostly associated with research or specialized assessments of top athletes, and have not been used in clinical settings. As far we are aware this is the first study using an HHD to perform concentric measurement, so it is not possible to define clinical agreement values to assess the LOA calculated in this paper. Instead, the LOA have been calculated to provide useful benchmarks for future research and a subjective analysis of the LOA is provided.

For elbow flexion, the LOA for peak torque are -11.6 and 13.5 Nm and for work are -24.1 and 26.0 J. The LOA of the peak torque angle are -21 and 69° which is unacceptable as a valid measurement of peak torque angle.

Eliminating participants who generate torque greater than 50 Nm, any tests with speed greater than 100°/s, and the first run of all the Biodex results improves the LOA of all the parameters. They are: -7.0 and 9.9Nm for peak torques, -15 and 53° for peak torque angle, and -12.4 and 16.2 J for work in elbow flexion.

Considering that the maximum peak torque is approximately 50 Nm, the LOA are approximately ±20% of the range of measurement, therefore we suggest that the use of IRL-HHD in muscle strength assessment provides the clinician with at least 5 additional scales above the MRC score of 5, assuming that the Biodex measurements are the accepted peak torques of the participants.

For knee extension, the LOA in all measurements show unacceptably large ranges. There is an obvious trend between mean strength and difference between the two devices, showing that the stronger the participant, the bigger the difference between the IRL-HHD and the Biodex measurements in peak torque. The LOA calculation with the proposed reduced dataset as discussed for elbow flexion are -23.1 and 28.7 Nm for peak torques, -16 and 41° for peak torque angle, and -13.1 and 41.0 J for total work. This means that for the knee extension test, the LOA of peak torque are approximately ±50% of the range of measurement, which is not a significant improvement over the conventional method.

Other factors that may affect the IRL-HHD assessments include: discomfort over the anterior tibial region because of the hard padding of the IRL-HHD force plate; the participants might be trying to control the speed; or they might think that the physiotherapist would not be able to control a maximal effort were they to exert it.

5. Conclusions

The new IRL-HHD has excellent intratester reliability, when used by an experienced user on healthy adults, for measuring peak torque and total work for elbow flexion and knee extension. Therefore, the device and the associated test protocols described in this paper can be used to measure these two physical attributes. The device is only reliable for determining peak torque angle if the mean of at least three repeated measurements is taken.

The LOA between the IRL-HHD and the isokinetic dynamometer are only reasonable for measuring elbow flexion peak torque and work. There were no agreements for peak torque and work of knee extension and peak torque angles of both elbow flexion and knee extension. Therefore, the IRL-HHD cannot be used on large muscle groups, such as the quadriceps, of healthy adults. The LOA also imply that the strength of the assessor using the IRL-HHD constrains the maximum forces that may be exerted by the subject, similar to the constraints reported for other hand-held isometric dynamometers.

The results obtained with the IRL-HHD cannot be compared with those obtained with an isokinetic dynamometer. However, since it has excellent intratester reliability, it can be used to compare strengths of different subjects or of one subject at different times, if used by the same assessor with the same test protocol.

6. Potential usage and future work

Recently, a study has been published on the reliability of shoulder assessment in patients with shoulder pain using the IRL-HHD (Cadogan et al. (2011)). These results show a good to excellent reliability of the IRL-HHD in practice.

The ability of measuring simultaneously the orientation of the device and the force imposed on the force plate may lead to many other potential usages. Other applications in which the IRL-HHD could be used include:

- In an isometric setting, the device can provide additional feedback on the tested angle. An audible angle warning feature can help the therapist to keep the joint within a pre-defined range, making the assessment more reliable (Sole et al. (2010), Hanna et al. (2010), Fulcher et al. (2010)).
- In the above described study of shoulder assessment (Cadogan et al. (2011)), a standardized shoulder lateral abduction active end range measurement was introduced. Since the end range of the shoulder is dependent on the amount of force the clinician exerts, it is impossible to compare measurements made by different assessors. However, with the IRL-HHD, a pre-set force can be entered into the IRL-HHD and when the force exerted on the force pad reaches the pre-set level, the IRL-HHD gives an audible warning sound so that the clinician knows when to click a button on the IRL-HHD to record the angle measurement. This should alleviate the assessors' variable strength issue.
- For measuring joint stiffness. Stiffness is defined as the rate of change of force with respect to the rate of change of displacement. Since the IRL-HHD can measure force and angle simultaneously, it is ideal for measuring stiffness.

- Measurement of children's dynamic strengths, as children are generally weaker than clinicians. Children are often too small to fit the isokinetic machines, and it would be difficult to strap a young child to the Biodex machine. Children may not be as patient as adults and so a rapid assessment using the IRL-HHD could offer some advantages.
- In people with disability, where transferring patients in and out of the isokinetic dynamometer is difficult.
- In cases when it is impossible to restrain the patient to the machine e.g. in patients with spasticity.

Future work should concentrate on developing and carrying out clinical trials for measuring the dynamic strength of people with injury or disability, small muscle groups in adult population or all muscle groups in children. For large muscle group assessments, additional fixtures to provide mechanical advantages for the assessors may be a solution for low-cost functional dynamic strength assessment tools.

7. Acknowledgements

This work was supported by the Foundation for Research Science and Technology, New Zealand (C08X0816). We thank Burwood Academy of Independent Living and the School of Physiotherapy, Otago University for their assistance in this research.

8. References

Andrews, A. (1991). Hand-held dynamometry for measuring muscle strength, *Journal of Human Muscle Performance* 1: 35–50.

Baltzopoulos, V. & Brodie, D. (1989). Isokinetic dynamometry. applications and limitations, *Sports Medicine (Auckland, N.Z.)* 8(2): 101–116. PMID: 2675256.

Bland, J. M. & Altman, D. G. (1986). Statistical methods for assessing agreement between two methods of clinical measurement, *Lancet* 1(8476): 307–310. PMID: 2868172.

Bland, J. M. & Altman, D. G. (2007). Agreement between methods of measurement with multiple observations per individual, *Journal of Biopharmaceutical Statistics* 17(4): 571.

Bohannon, R. W. & Andrews, A. W. (1987). Interrater reliability of Hand-Held dynamometry, *Physical Therapy* 67(6): 931 –933.

Cadogan, A., Laslett, M., Hing, W., McNair, P. & Williams, M. (2011). Reliability of a new hand-held dynamometer in measuring shoulder range of motion and strength, *Manual Therapy* 16(1): 97–101.

Clarkson, H. M. (2000). *Musculoskeletal assessment: joint range of motion and manual muscle strength*, Lippincott Williams & Wilkins.

Cuthbert, S. C. & Goodheart, G. J. (2007). On the reliability and validity of manual muscle testing: a literature review, *Chiropractic & Osteopathy* 15(1): 4.

Drouin, J. M., Valovich-mcLeod, T. C., Shultz, S. J., Gansneder, B. M. & Perrin, D. H. (2004). Reliability and validity of the biodex system 3 pro isokinetic dynamometer velocity, torque and position measurements, *European Journal of Applied Physiology* 91(1): 22–29.

Edwards, R. H. & McDonnell, M. (1974). Hand-held dynamometer for evaluating voluntary-muscle function, *Lancet* 2(7883): 757–758. PMID: 4143018.

Fleiss, J. L. (1986). *The Design and Analysis of Clinical Experiments*, 1 edn, John Wiley & Sons.

Frese, E., Brown, M. & Norton, B. J. (1987). Clinical reliability of manual muscle testing, *Physical Therapy* 67(7): 1072 –1076.

Fulcher, M. L., Hanna, C. M. & Raina Elley, C. (2010). Reliability of handheld dynamometry in assessment of hip strength in adult male football players, *Journal of Science and Medicine in Sport* 13(1): 80–84.

Hanna, C. M., Fulcher, M. L., Elley, C. R. & Moyes, S. A. (2010). Normative values of hip strength in adult male association football players assessed by handheld dynamometry, *Journal of Science and Medicine in Sport* 13(3): 299–303.

Harlaar, J., Roebroeck, M. E. & Lankhorst, G. J. (1996). Computer-assisted hand-held dynamometer: low-cost instrument for muscle function assessment in rehabilitation medicine, *Medical & Biological Engineering & Computing* 34(5): 329–335.

Hyde, S. A., Goddard, C. M. & Scott, O. M. (1983). The myometer: the development of a clinical tool, *Physiotherapy* 69(12): 424–427. PMID: 6665080.

Janssen, J. C. & Le-Ngoc, L. (2009). Intratester reliability and validity of concentric measurements using a new Hand-Held dynamometer, *Archives of Physical Medicine and Rehabilitation* 90(9): 1541–1547.

Kannus, P. (1994). Isokinetic evaluation of muscular performance: implications for muscle testing and rehabilitation, *International Journal of Sports Medicine* 15 Suppl 1: S11–18. PMID: 8157377.

Li, R. C., Jasiewicz, J. M., Middleton, J., Condie, P., Barriskill, A., Hebnes, H. & Purcell, B. (2006). The development, validity, and reliability of a manual muscle testing device with integrated limb position sensors, *Archives of Physical Medicine and Rehabilitation* 87(3): 411–417.

Lund, H., Søndergaard, K., Zachariassen, T., Christensen, R., Bülow, P., Henriksen, M., Bartels, E. M., Danneskiold-Samsøe, B. & Bliddal, H. (2005). Learning effect of isokinetic measurements in healthy subjects, and reliability and comparability of biodex and lido dynamometers, *Clinical Physiology and Functional Imaging* 25(2): 75–82.

Martin, H., Yule, V., Syddall, H., Dennison, E., Cooper, C. & Aihie Sayer, A. (2006). Is Hand-Held dynamometry useful for the measurement of quadriceps strength in older people? a comparison with the gold standard biodex dynamometry, *Gerontology* 52(3): 154–159.

Mital, A., Kopardekar, P. & Motorwala, A. (1995). Isokinetic pull strengths in the vertical plane: effects of speed and arm angle, *Clinical Biomechanics* 10(2): 110–112.

Osternig, L. R. (1986). Isokinetic dynamometry: implications for muscle testing and rehabilitation, *Exercise and Sport Sciences Reviews* 14: 45–80. PMID: 3525192.

Petty, N. (2011). *Neuromusculoskeletal examination and assessment : a handbook for therapists*, 4th ed. edn, Churchill Livingstone/Elsevier, Edinburgh ; New York.

Roebroeck, M. E., Harlaar, J. & Lankhorst, G. J. (1998). Reliability assessment of isometric knee extension measurements with a computer-assisted hand-held dynamometer, *Archives of Physical Medicine and Rehabilitation* 79(4): 442–448. PMID: 9552112.

Sole, G., Wright, L., Wassinger, C., Higgs, C., Hansson, M., Johansson, S. & Todd, N. (2010). Reliability of hand held dynamometric strength testing in people with diabetes/chronic conditions, *New Zealand Journal of Physiotherapy* 38 (2): 52–55.

Stark, T., Walker, B., Phillips, J., Fejer, R. & Beck, R. (2011). Hand-held dynamometry correlation with the gold standard isokinetic dynamometry: A systematic review, *Physical Medicine and Rehabilitation* 3(5): 472–479.

van der Ploeg, R. J., Oosterhuis, H. J. & Reuvekamp, J. (1984). Measuring muscle strength, *Journal of Neurology* 231(4): 200–203. PMID: 6512574.

Wikholm, J. B. & Bohannon, R. W. (1991). Hand-held dynamometer measurements: Tester strength makes a difference, *The Journal of Orthopaedic and Sports Physical Therapy* 13(4): 191–198. PMID: 18796845.

5

Functional Recovery and Muscle Properties After Stroke: A Preliminary Longitudinal Study

Astrid Horstman, Arnold de Haan, Manin Konijnenbelt, Thomas Janssen and Karin Gerrits
VU University Amsterdam, The Netherlands

1. Introduction

Almost all patients with stroke experience a certain degree of functional recovery within the first six months after stroke. Most recovery of motor and functional performance is seen in the first month after stroke (Gray et al., 1990; Duncan et al., 1992, 1994; Jorgensen et al., 1995; Horgan & Finn, 1997; Kong et al., 2011) but improvement may continue as long as 6-12 months after stroke (Bonita & Beaglehole, 1988). Verheyden et al. (2008) observed most improvement for trunk, arm, leg and functional recovery from 1 week to 1 month after stroke and then to a lesser extent between 1 and 3 months after stroke. Only small, not statistically significant changes could be seen between 3 and 6 months after stroke, indicating that a "plateau phase" was already reached at 3 months after stroke. Further improvement after 6 months can be expected but is mostly limited (Mayo et al., 1999; Hendricks et al., 2002; Desrosiers et al., 2003; Kwakkel et al., 2004). Six months after stroke, only 60% of people with initial hemiparesis have achieved functional independence in simple activities of daily living such as toileting and walking short distances (Mayo et al., 1999; Patel et al., 2000). However, improvements in activities of daily living may continue despite stable deficits at the level of impairment. This is suggestive of further behavioral adaptation or compensation. Rehabilitation is devoted to enlarge and precipitate this functional recovery in order to improve quality of life after stroke (Gresham et al., 1995). Therefore, rehabilitation programs adapted to objectives as allowed by the state of the neuromuscular system are important.

Many daily activities, especially locomotion, require sufficient function of thigh muscles. A number of studies reported that lower extremity muscles are weaker in patients with stroke compared to healthy controls (Newham & Hsiao, 2001; Bohannon, 2007b; Sullivan et al., 2007; Horstman et al., 2008). Furthermore, the inability to generate normal amounts of force has been suggested to be the major limitation of physical activity (Mercier & Bourbonnais, 2004; Ada et al., 2006). More specific, intrinsic strength capacity as well as the ability to maximally activate the knee extensors correlate strongly with functional performance (daily activities) in patients with stroke (Bohannon, 1988, 1989; Corrigan & Bohannon, 2001; Kim & Eng, 2003; Bohannon, 2007b; Patterson et al., 2007; Horstman et al., 2008). In addition, a recent study showed a significant association between paretic lower limb strength and balance both *cross-sectionally* in *acute* patients with stroke as well as *longitudinally* in *post-acute* patients (van Nes et al., 2009).

Besides a reduction in maximal muscle strength, the ability to generate torque as fast as possible, is also impaired after stroke (Horstman et al., 2010; Bohannon & Walsh, 1992; Gerrits et al., 2009). Rate of torque development is an important determinant of e.g. risk of falling and (again) for controlling balance (Shigematsu et al., 2006; Pijnappels et al., 2008). Recent work from our group has shown lower maximal rates of torque development during electrically stimulated (Horstman et al., 2010; Gerrits et al., 2009) as well as during voluntary (Horstman et al., 2010) contractions of the paretic and non-paretic knee-extensors. Decreased ability to rapidly develop knee extension torque contributes more to lower walking speed after stroke than does maximal strength (Pohl et al., 2002).

In summary, there is clear evidence that difficulties in executing daily tasks in patients with stroke are related to both impaired strength and speed of paretic and/or non-paretic muscles. Nevertheless, most studies are performed at one point in time (Kim & Eng, 2003; Mercier & Bourbonnais, 2004; Ada et al., 2006; Bohannon, 2007b; Patterson et al., 2007; Horstman et al., 2008). It is not fully elucidated whether the improvements in functional performance at the activity level of patients with stroke during rehabilitation relate to changes in specific contractile function of the thigh muscles. Therefore, the present study reports on *longitudinal* changes in functional performance in a group of patients with stroke during the first year after stroke. Furthermore, it is determined whether these changes relate to alterations in strength and speed characteristics of the paretic and non-paretic thigh muscles and voluntary activation capacity of patients with stroke.

2. Methods

2.1 Subjects

A total number of fourteen patients were included in the study. Patients (characteristics: see Table 1), all with first-ever stroke and a hemiparesis of the lower extremity, entered the study on average 3.5 months after stroke and 2 months after admission in the rehabilitation centre (t=0). Data on muscle function in relation to functional performance of these patients at t=0 are reported elsewhere (Horstman et al., 2008). They were invited for measurements again 3 (n=8), 6 (n=5) and 12 (n=3) months after the first measurement (follow-up (F)1, F2 and F3 respectively). Because of drop-out of a number of subjects, data will be largely descriptive. Before participation, each subject was thoroughly informed about the procedures, completed a health questionnaire and signed an informed consent.

The exclusion criteria were medical complications (such as unstable cardiovascular problems), severe cognitive and/or communicative problems preventing understanding verbal instructions or limiting performance of the requested tasks (e.g. aphasia, hemineglect) and contra-indications for electrical stimulation (unstable epilepsy, cancer, skin abnormalities and pacemaker). The project carried the approval of the institutional review board (Medical Ethical Committee) of the VU University Medical Centre, Amsterdam, The Netherlands.

Subject no.	Gender	Age (yrs)	Weight (kg)	Height (cm)	Time after stroke (days)	Time after admission (days)	Side of lesion (Left/ Right)	Ischaemic/ Hemorrhage	Last measurement
1	Male	65	70	172	189	29	R	I	F3
2	Male	61	89	172	84	67	L	H	F3
3	Male	61	80	182	52	76	L	I	F3
4	Male	52	79	172	87	55	L	H	F2
5	Male	55	81	177	167	145	R	I	F2
6	Male	56	80	168	77	41	L	I	F1
7	Female	26	63	170	110	52	R	I	F1
8	Female	62	60	168	55	61	R	I	F1
9	Female	61	40	150	123	76	L	H	t=0
10	Male	57	69	180	170	70	R	I	t=0
11	Female	64	74	170	117	90	L	I	t=0
12	Male	45	80	190	79	35	R	H	t=0
13	Male	67	100	190	157	114	R	H	t=0
14	Male	58	83	178	56	29	R	I	t=0

Table 1. Subject characteristics.

2.2 Experimental set-up

Body function and activity-participation level were assessed with different clinical tests ('functional performance' tests). In addition, muscle function characteristics of the knee-extensors and -flexors were assessed in both limbs. The measurements were spread over four different days with at least one day of rest in between.

2.3 Experimental procedures

2.3.1 Functional performance tests

The following tests were performed by the subjects under supervision of a physiotherapist (except for the Rivermead Mobility Index, which was carried out by one of the researchers):

- *Berg Balance Scale (BBS)* assesses sitting and standing balance and exists of 14 test-items, scored on an ordinal 5-point scale (0-4). It gives an estimation of the chance that patients with stroke will fall (Berg et al., 1989, 1992, 1995).
- *Brunnstrom Fugl-Meyer (FM), lower extremity,* is a test for evaluation of patellar, knee flexor and Achilles reflexes, flexor and extensor synergies, isolated movements of knee flexor and ankle dorsal flexor function and normal reflex activity of the quadriceps and triceps surae muscles in the paretic lower limb hemiplegic patients (Fugl-Meyer et al., 1975). Maximal possible score is 34.
- *Rivermead Mobility Index (RMI)* comprises a series of 14 questions and one direct observation, and covers a range of activities from turning over in bed to running. It is a measure of mobility disability which concentrates on body mobility (Collen et al., 1991).
- *Timed "get-up-and-*go" test (TUG) requires patients to stand up from a chair, walk 3m, turn around, return, and sit down again. Time to fulfil this test is measured (Podsiadlo & Richardson, 1991). The shorter the time needed to do this test, the better; for all other tests applies the higher the score, the better.

- *10 meter walk test (10m)* is performed at comfortable (self selected) walking speed by patients who are able to walk independent with or without mobility aid and/or orthesis. Time to walk 10m is measured and averaged over three trials (Smith & Baer, 1999). Then, the speed is calculated (10m divided by the average time to walk that 10m).
- *Motricity Index (MI)* evaluates the arbitrary movement activity and maximum isometric muscle force. Possible scores are 0-9-14-19-25-33 at each of the three parts of the test for lower extremities (Demeurisse et al., 1980; Collin & Wade, 1990; Cameron & Bohannon, 2000).
- *Functional Ambulation Categories-score* (*FAC*) evaluates the measure of independence of walking of the patient. Categories are scored on a six-point scale (0-5) (Holden *et al.*, 1984, 1986).

2.3.2 Force measurements

The procedures for the measurements as well as the calculation of variables are described in detail elsewhere (Horstman et al., 2008). Briefly, maximal voluntary and electrically evoked isometric torques of the knee extensors and maximal voluntary isometric torques of the knee flexors were measured while subjects were seated on a custom built Lower EXtremity System (LEXS) (Horstman et al., 2008). The lower leg was strapped tightly to a force transducer just above the ankle by means of a cuff at a knee flexion angle of 60° (0° = full extension). Electrical stimulation, used for the knee extensors only, was applied via two surface electrodes placed over the quadriceps muscles with a computer-controlled constant current stimulator (Digitimer DSH7, Digitimer Ltd., Welwyn Garden City, UK).

2.3.3 Familiarization session

During the familiarization session, measurements were performed with the non-paretic lower limb to check whether the instructions were understood by the subject. After a warming-up (existing of 5 submaximal contractions) subjects were trained to perform maximal isometric knee flexion (MVCf) and extension (MVCe) contractions and fast voluntary knee extensions. Subsequently, the subjects were familiarized with electrical stimulation. During the follow-up measurements, no familiarization session was performed.

2.3.4 Muscle strength and speed

Subjects were asked to maximally generate isometric knee extensions for 3-4 s to determine MVCe. Alternately, MVCfs were performed, as described in Horstman et al. (2008). Thereafter, subjects were asked to perform knee extensions as fast as possible (Horstman et al., 2008) with the command: 3, 2, 1 GO! They were encouraged to reach a peak force of at least 70% of their MVC and were not allowed to make a countermovement (flexion) or have pretension before the fast extension (de Ruiter et al., 2004). The same measurements as performed with the paretic lower limb (PL) were repeated with the non-paretic lower limb (NL), carried out on a separate day. Control subjects just performed one session, with the right leg only.

2.3.5 Triplet stimulation and voluntary activation

A modified super-imposed stimulation technique was used in which electrically evoked triplets (pulse train of three rectangular 200 μs pulses applied at 300 Hz) were used to establish the subjects' capacity to voluntarily activate their muscles (Kooistra et al., 2005). Measurements started with PL in a knee angle of 60° knee flexion. First, stimulation current was increased until supramaximal stimulation was ensured. Next, subjects underwent measurements consisting of a triplet superimposed on the plateau of the force signal of the MVC. Subsequently, these measurements were performed with NL.

2.4 Data analysis of muscle function

MVC torque (Nm) was determined as the peak force from the force plateau multiplied by the external moment arm. MVCe and MVCf were assessed. *Maximal rate of torque development* was defined as the steepest slope of torque development during fast voluntary contractions (MRTDvol) (de Ruiter et al., 2004) and during a pulse train of 80 ms, 300 Hz (MRTDstim). MRTDvol was normalized to MVCe torque in order to correct for the number of parallel muscle fibers ('muscle thickness') to get a fair comparison of contractile speed of muscles between different subjects independent of absolute maximal torques. MRTDstim was therefore expressed as a percentage of 150 Hz torque (obtained at the same stimulation intensity as the 300 Hz pulse train).

Voluntary activation is defined as the completeness of skeletal muscle activation during voluntary contractions and was calculated by means of a modified interpolated twitch technique (Kooistra et al., 2005). *Voluntary activation (%) = [1 – (superimposed triplet/rest triplet)] * 100.* Here the superimposed triplet is the force increment during a maximal contraction at the time of stimulation and the control triplet is that evoked in the relaxed muscle (Shield & Zhou, 2004). Supramaximal *triplet torque* of the relaxed muscle is used as a measure for the maximal (intrinsic) torque capacity of the knee extensors, independent of voluntary activation.

Spearman rank correlations were calculated between changes (Δ, between t=0 and F2) in scores at the tests of functional performance and changes in the 6 muscle variables (MVCe, MVCf, MRTDvol, MRTDstim, triplet and voluntary activation). For the differences over time, shown in Table 2, a Friedman test was used.

3. Results

Not all subjects participated in follow-up sessions. The most important reason given was that travelling to the testing site was too time-consuming. Some experienced the measurements (especially the electrical stimulation and the duration of the experiments) as too uncomfortable. Other patients missed the follow-up measurements due to severe illness. One patient decided to spend the winter abroad. Moreover, data were not complete for some of the patients due to unreliability, e.g. concentration problems (one subject dozed off a few times during the measurements), no force plateau during the MVCs or subjects did not reach 90% of their MVC during the familiarization session. Therefore, the data will be mainly descriptive and hardly any statistical analyses were performed.

3.1 Functional performance

Figure 1 shows the course of the scores of the subjects with stroke at two important (see below, Table 4) tests of functional performance, namely the BBS, a measure of ability-activity level, and at the FM, an impairment (bodily functions) measure developed to assess physical recovery after stroke (Sanford et al., 1993). Because the outcome of most tests of functional performance seemed to plateau at F2 and because F3 values could only be obtained in three subjects, mean values of the five subjects assessed until F2 are presented in Table 2. Data in this table are expressed as median and 1st and 3rd quartile. Overall, the data of the functional performance tests show improvement (except for MI) during the follow-up period.

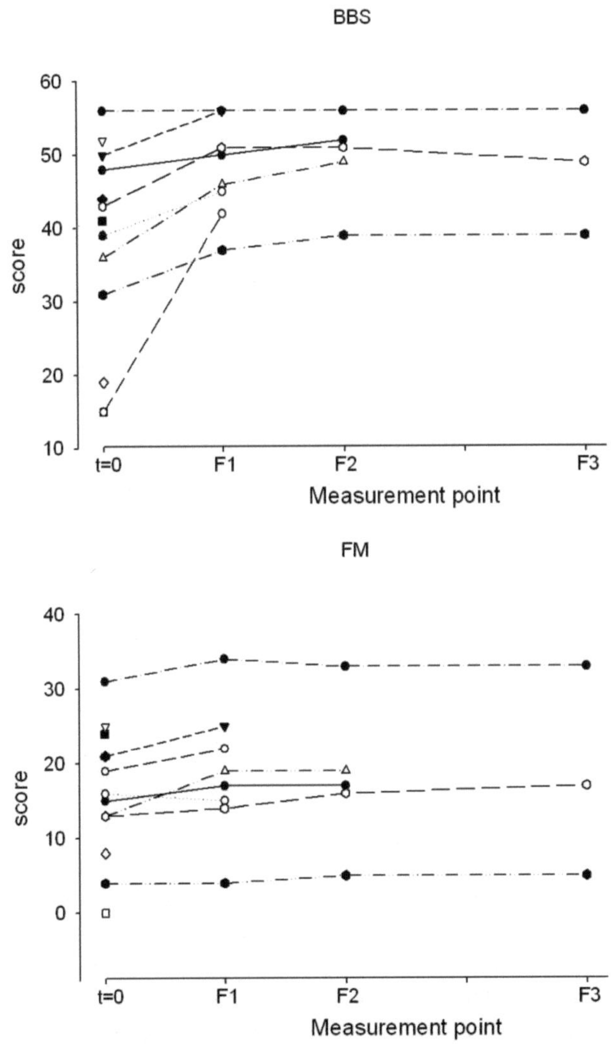

Fig. 1. Course of all individual scores at the Berg Balance Scale (BBS) and Brunnstrom Fugl-Meyer, lower extremity (FM) at 4 measuring times (t=0, F1, F2, F3). Note that t=0 is on average 3.5 months after stroke.

	t=0	F1	F2
BBS	43 (36-48)	50 (46-51)*	51 (49-52)*
MI	42 (39-47)	61 (42-64)	61 (53-61)
FAC	4 (3-4)	5 (4-5)*	5 (5-5)*
RMI	8 (7-8)	13 (12-13)*	13 (12-13)*
FM	13 (13-15)	17(14-19)^	17 (16-10)*
10m (m/s)	0.28 (0.23-0.39))	0.36 (0.35-0.47)^	0.35 (0.30-0.53)*
TUG (s)	43.5 (34.7-49.0)	34.0 (34.0-41.0)	30.1(20.8-38.0)^

* significant improvement (p<0.05) compared with t=0
^ trend (p<0.1) compared with t=0

Table 2. Median values and 1st and 3rd quartiles for the Berg Balance Scale (BBS), Motricity Index (MI), Functional Ambulation Categories-score (FAC), Rivermead Mobility Index (RMI), Brunnstrom Fugl-Meyer (FM), 10 meter walk test (10m) and Timed "get-up-and-go" test (TUG) at the 3 measurement points 3.5 months after stroke (t=0) and during follow-up (F)1 and F2 for the five subjects who participated at these three measurement points (n= 5).

3.2 Muscle variables

Data were not complete for reasons explained earlier. Furthermore, it is a general experience that subjects, knowing that a superimposed stimulation will be performed, anticipate upon stimulation and perform less when compared with MVC without stimulation. To minimize this effect, which influences the activation results, only data were used when MVCs with superimposed stimulation were more than 90% of their highest attempt. Therefore, variables of muscle functions in Table 3 show missing values. The zero values are values from subjects who did perform the measurements but were not able to generate force with their paretic lower limb.

There was a substantial variation between subjects with respect to the outcome of the muscle variables at the start of the study (t=0) as well as with respect to the changes in these variables over time (Table 3).

3.3 Correlations between changes in functional performance and muscle function

Table 4 shows the potential relevant correlations (n=4 or 5) with $|\rho|>0.7$ between changes (Δ, i.e., MVCe at F2 minus MVCe at t=0) in scores at tests of functional performance and changes in muscle variables. Figure 2 shows the five significant correlations namely the correlations between ΔMVCf of PL and Δ10m (ρ=0.99, p=0.002, n=5), between ΔMRTDstim of PL and ΔFM (ρ=0.99, p=0.01, n=4), between Δtriplet of PL and ΔFM (ρ=0.90, p=0.04, n=5), between Δtriplet of PL and ΔRMI (ρ=0.92, p=0.03, n=5), and between ΔMVCf of NL and ΔBBS (ρ=0.92, p=0.03, n=5).

4. Discussion

A considerable improvement was found in de scores at the tests of functional performance, especially up to F2. In general also the muscle variables improved over time. Changes in muscle variables of the 5 subjects that were measured at t=0, F1 and F2 were shown to correlate with improvements in tests of functional performance during the first 9 months after stroke.

	Subject	PL t=0	PL F1	PL F2	NL t=0	NL F1	NL F2
MVCe (Nm)	**1**	0	0	0	149	125	145
	2	35	30	63	101	109	130
	3	171	149	186	250	245	255
	4	82	105	132	145	174	156
	5	64	107	137	162	171	246
MVCf (Nm)	**1**	0	0	0	35	13	53
	2	1	0	8	39	60	68
	3	50	51	73	90	92	88
	4	0	0	0	68	60	62
	5	0	0	0	54	71	101
MRTDvol (% · ms^{-1})	**1**	0.00	0.00	0.00	4.16	5.93	5.83
	2	2.03	-	2.59	5.74	-	4.70
	3	7.08	10.53	8.62	9.29	6.44	3.51
	4	3.30	2.87	3.82	4.69	3.77	3.51
	5	5.19	6.27	7.11	9.34	7.92	8.30
MRTDstim (% · ms^{-1})	**1**	10.31	15.51	14.24	12.77	13.24	14.24
	2	5.46	-	11.35	13.78	16.40	16.88
	3	16.77	19.03	21.22	26.28	37.97	30.00
	4	14.13	9.07	-	14.39	13.14	-
	5	9.07	12.07	19.68	8.67	11.44	19.43
Triplet torque (Nm)	**1**	41	42	48	84	84	94
	2	29	-	44	50	52	42
	3	110	101	112	113	112	109
	4	82	104	96	110	115	100
	5	75	90	103	110	115	100
VA (%)	**1**	-	-	-	70	55	69
	2	16	-	57	75	-	85
	3	73	75	79	88	93	91
	4	64	55	55	68	85	73
	5	42	59	75	75	81	80

Table 3. Data on muscle variables for 5 subjects who were measured during the first measurement (t=0) and 3 and 6 months thereafter (F1, F2 respectively) for the non-paretic (NL) and paretic lower limb (PL). Maximal voluntary extension (MVCe) and flexion (MVCf) torque, maximal rate of torque development during voluntary (MRTDvol) and electrically evoked contractions (MRTDstim), triplet torque and voluntary activation (VA).

		BBS	FM	RMI	10m (m/s)	FAC	TUG (s)	MI
PL	MVCe	-	0.843^	0.861^	-	-	-	0.832^
	MVCf	-	-	-	0.985*	-	-	-
	MRTDvol	-	0.750	-	-	-	-	-
	MRTDstim	0.736	0.990*	0.860	-	-	-	0.815
	Triplet	0.827^	0.897*	0.923*	-	-	-	-
	VA	0.710	-	-	-	-	-	-
NL	MVCe	0.745	N.A.	0.833^	-	-	-	-
	MVCf	0.922*	N.A.	-	-	-	-	-
	MRTDvol	-	N.A.	-	-	-	-0.881	-
	MRTDstim	-	N.A.	0.719	-	-	-	0.732
	Triplet	-	N.A.	-	-	-	-	-
	VA	-	N.A.	0.742	-	-	-	-

* significant ($p<0.05$) correlation, ^ trend ($p<0.1$)

Table 4. Correlation coefficients between changes (between t=0 and F2) in scores at tests of functional performance and changes in muscle variables for the non-paretic (NL) and paretic lower limb (PL) of 5 subjects. Berg Balance Scale (BBS), Motricity Index (MI), Functional Ambulation Categories-score (FAC), Rivermead Mobility Index (RMI) and Brunnstrom Fugl-Meyer (FM), Timed "get-up-and-go" test (TUG) and 10 meter walk test (10m). Maximal voluntary extension (MVCe) and flexion (MVCf) torque, maximal rate of torque development during voluntary (MRTDvol) and electrically evoked contractions (MRTDstim), triplet torque and voluntary activation (VA).

4.1 Functional performance

From the 5 subjects we followed until F2, subject 1 scored the lowest values of all subjects (n=14) that took part in the study at t=0 at all variables of the paretic lower limb (Table 3), whereas subject 3 scored the best. The actual improvement in the Timed "get-up-and-go" test (TUG) between t=0 and F2 may be even greater than presented in Table 2. Subject 1 was not able to perform the TUG at t=0, but during F1 that subject was able to do the TUG in 81 s. Nevertheless, the score of this subject could not be used, since the improvement could not be calculated due to the missing value at t=0. This same subject 1 scored 9 on the Motricity Index (MI) at t=0 but 0 at F1 and F2. Moreover, subject 3 achieved the maximal score of 100 at MI for all three measurement points and only one subject improved between F1 and F2 at this test. This may explain why we found no significant improvement over time for MI in the five subjects who came for these 2 follow-ups.

An improvement of 7%, from 45 to 52% of maximum attainable recovery (n=8) at the Fugl-Meyer Lower Extremity test (FM) was found from ~3.5 months (t=0) to half a year (F1) after stroke (n=8) (Figure 2). For FAC a significant increase from 68 to 88% was found and for MI 47 to 53% (not significant) (Table 2). Kwakkel et al. (2004) similarly observed an improvement from about 62% to 65% at the FM (n=101), 51 to 59% at the FAC and 58 to 59% at the MI during the first half year after stroke. Both the present results and those of Kwakkel et al. (2004) show that most improvement took place within the first 3 months until half year after stroke, as was also found by others (Wade & Hewer, 1987; Jorgeson et al., 1995).

4.2 Muscle variables

As would be expected after hemiparetic stroke, PL scored consistently lower than NL on the muscle variables (voluntary extension and flexion torque, triplet torque, voluntary activation and maximal rate of voluntary torque development). Variable results in changes in muscle characteristics were found per subject between t=0 and F2 (Table 3). Also in literature there are different results. Carin-Levy et al. (2006) reported, in line with our results, no significant change over time in the strength and muscle mass of both paretic and non-paretic (arm and) leg muscle during the first 6 months after stroke. However, Newham and Hsiao (2001) did observe increased strength throughout the first half year after stroke, while activation failure remained constant. Andrews et al. (2003) showed an increase in both PL and NL knee extensor strength from admission (~2 wk post stroke) to discharge (~4 wk post stroke). So, there are no consistent data indicating that muscle variables improve after stroke.

The main limitation of our study is the small sample size at F2 and F3. Although all new patients with stroke in the rehabilitation centre were examined by physicians, a large number were ineligible for our study, because they had severe cognitive and/or communicative problems, medical complications, no hemiparesis of the lower extremity or, conversely, were too heavily paralyzed and had a previous stroke. A considerable number of patients were not willing to participate (or in case of follow-ups to continue), mainly due to their changed life after stroke and/or the intensity of the protocol. Around half of the eligible patients completed the entire protocol (4 measurement days) at t=0. The scores of stroke severity of our patients (FAC median and quartiles 4 (2.25-4)) confirmed that we managed to recruit a very wide a range of patients with stroke at t=0, but this contributed to the difficulty in statistics, besides the great drop-out of patients during the follow-ups. However, studies with smaller samples sizes than ours have detected significant changes in muscle strength over time in NL (Harris et al., 2001) and PL compared to control (Newham & Hsiao, 2001). Thus, it is likely that, if changes in the thigh muscles of our patients had occurred, these must have been small.

4.3 Correlation between muscle variables and functional performance

The severity of post stroke paresis is related to a person's ability to perform functional tasks; Others found correlations between lower limb isometric knee extension strength and functional performance, like gait distance (Bohannon, 1989) and speed (Bohannon, 1989; Bohannon & Walsh, 1991, 1992; Horstman et al., 2008), sit-to-stand (Bohannon, 2007a; Horstman et al., 2008), transfers (Bohannon, 1988), stair climbing (Bohannon & Walsh, 1991) and balance (Horstman et al., 2008). The new aspect in this study is that we wanted to investigate whether *changes* in functional performance during the first 9 months after stroke related to changes in muscle characteristics.

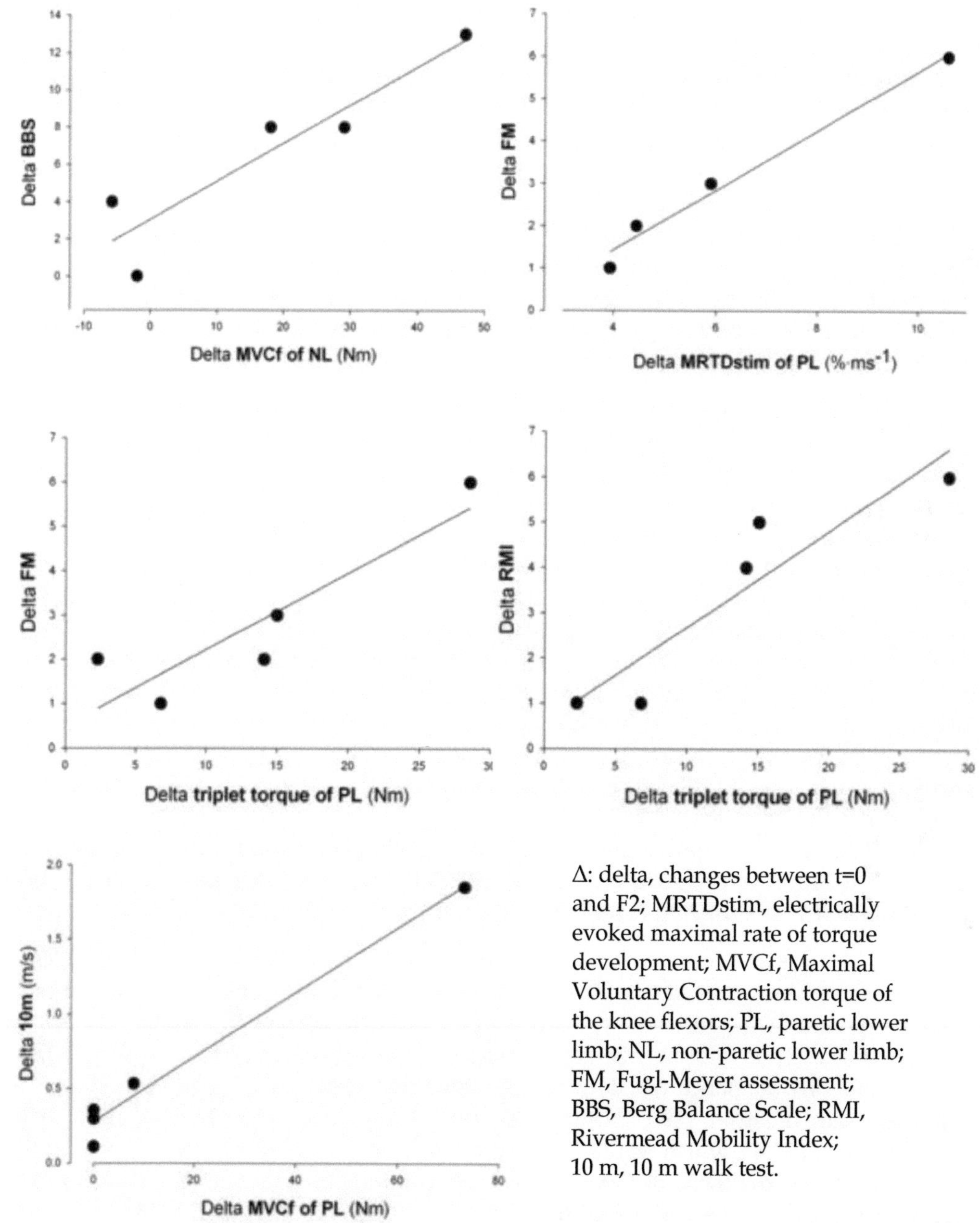

Δ: delta, changes between t=0 and F2; MRTDstim, electrically evoked maximal rate of torque development; MVCf, Maximal Voluntary Contraction torque of the knee flexors; PL, paretic lower limb; NL, non-paretic lower limb; FM, Fugl-Meyer assessment; BBS, Berg Balance Scale; RMI, Rivermead Mobility Index; 10 m, 10 m walk test.

Fig. 2. Correlations between ΔMRTDstim of PL and ΔFM (ρ=0.99, p=0.01, n=4), between Δtriplet of PL and ΔFM (ρ=0.90, p=0.04, n=5), between Δtriplet of PL and ΔRMI (ρ=0.92, p=0.03, n=5), between ΔMVCf of NL and ΔBBS (ρ=0.92, p=0.03, n=5) and between ΔMVCf of PL and Δ10m (ρ=0.99, p=0.002, n=5).

Most relations were found within subjects between changes in muscle variables of PL and changes in scores at the BBS, a sitting and standing balance measure and the FM, an impairment measure developed to assess physical recovery after stroke (Sanford et al., 1993). Moreover, changes in flexor strength are positively related with changes in the 10m walking speed, which means the more increase in hamstring strength, the bigger the increase in walking speed. In our cross-sectional study (Horstman et al., 2008) strong significant correlations were found between muscle variables of both PL and NL and various tests of functional performance. However, in the present study if we look within subjects, we hardly see any correlations between changes in muscle variables of NL and changes in scores at the functional performance tests over time. This indicates that longitudinal data are essential to gain the required information regarding which (muscle) variables should be trained to induce improvements in functional performance, because cross-sectional data are not exclusive enough.

A question that remains to be answered is what may have caused the improvements in functional recovery? It is suggested that functional gains experienced by patients with stroke are primarily attributable to spontaneous recovery (changes over time that occur naturally) of functional performance of which eighty percent occurs within six months after the onset of stroke (Lind, 1982). Others state that there is some recovery between 1 and 6 months in almost all acute patients with stroke (Wade & Hewer, 1987) and that at 6 months 60% of people with initial hemiparesis have achieved functional independence in daily activities such as toileting and walking short distances (Mayo et al., 1999; Patel et al., 2000.) To facilitate neuroplasticity and cortical reorganization, it would be interesting to also investigate sensory stimulation in future studies with patients with stroke (Nudo et al., 1996; Johansson, 2000) since sensory impairments of all modalities are common after stroke (Carey, 1995). Moreover, sensory deficits are associated with the degree of weakness and the degree of stroke severity related to mobility, independence in activities of daily living, and recovery (De Haart et al., 2004; Lin, 2005). Addressing sensory deficits that accompany muscle weakness may improve impaired processing of afferent signals which in turn may contribute to improved muscle activation, gait patterns, and responses to perturbation during gait and stance (El-Abd & Ibrahim, 1994).

Secondary changes as a result of stroke could be expected in skeletal muscle, e.g. changes in myofiber type (De Deyne et al., 2004) or number and size of motor units. The latter is already reported in the second week after stroke onset (Jorgensen & Jacobsen, 2001). For instance, a change in muscle fiber composition, characterized by selective type II fiber atrophy and predominance of (slow twitch, oxidative) type I fibers has been shown in paretic muscles (Edstrom, 1970; Scelsi et al., 1984; Dietz et al., 1986; Dattola et al., 1993; Hachisuka et al., 1997), which would lead to concomitant changes in contractile speed of the muscle fibers towards those of slow muscles. We can imagine that such a change in fiber type composition can be combated, for instance by training, during the first year after stroke, so that muscle speed characteristics can be restored. Bohannon concludes in his review (Bohannon, 2007b) that resistance training programs are effective at increasing strength in patients who have experienced a stroke but there is no clear evidence for the effect of strength training on functional activities after stroke (Morris et al., 2004). Main results of Saunders' review (Saunders et al., 2004) include only 4 strength training trials (Inaba et al., 1973; Kim et al., 2001; Ouellette et al., 2004; Winstein et al., 2004) and lack nonexercise attention controls, long-term training and follow up. Strength measures were reported to improve after resistance training, albeit without clear benefits for functional performance (e.g. gait speed) (Saunders et al., 2004). Therefore, in addition, the strength training may be combined with task-specific functional training (Sullivan et al., 2006; Hubbard et al., 2009), because it has "the potential to drive brain reorganization toward more optimal functional performance" (Shepherd, 2001). When muscles are weak, isometric contractions can be used in the early stages of rehabilitation as a means of improving the muscle's ability to contract. However, once muscle strength reaches a certain threshold, exercises should be biomechanically similar to daily life actions in order to be trained to transfer increased force-generating ability into improved performance (Shepherd, 2001).

5. Conclusion

The (small) alterations in the muscle variables correlated well with the improvements in scores on tests of functional performance. Although the correlations do not necessarily imply causality, we think (intrinsic) muscle speed and strength are important variables which can potentially be prolific targets to improve during rehabilitation. It is therefore recommended to investigate the effects of strength training of the thigh muscles during at least the first 6 months after stroke. From such an intervention study on functional recovery it can be elucidated whether increasing strength and speed really improves functional performance.

6. References

Ada L, Dorsch S & Canning CG. (2006). Strengthening interventions increase strength and improve activity after stroke: a systematic review. *Australian Journal of Physiotherapy* 52(4):241-8

Andrews AW & Bohannon RW. (2003). Short-term recovery of limb muscle strength after acute stroke. *Archives of Physical Medicine and Rehabilitation* Jan;84(1):125-30

Berg K, Wood- Dauphinee S, Williams JI & Gayton D. (1989). Measuring balance in the elderly: preliminary development of an instrument. *Physiotherapy Canada* 41:304-311

Berg KO, Wood-Dauphinee SL & Williams JI. (1995). The Balance Scale: reliability assessment with elderly residents and patients with an acute stroke. *Scandinavian Journal of Rehabilitation Medicine* Mar;27(1):27-36

Berg KO, Wood-Dauphinee SL, Williams JI & Maki B. (1992). Measuring balance in the elderly: validation of an instrument. *Canadian Journal of Public Health* Jul-Aug;83 Suppl 2:S7-11

Bohannon RW. (1988). Determinants of transfer capacity in patients with hemiparesis. *Physiotherapy Canada* 40:236-239

Bohannon RW. (1989). Is the measurement of muscle strength appropriate in patients with brain lesions? A special communication. *Physical Therapy* Mar;69(3):225-36

Bohannon RW. (2007a). Knee extension strength and body weight determine sit-to-stand independence after stroke. *Physiotherapy: Theory and Practice* Sep-Oct;23(5):291-7

Bohannon RW. (2007b). Muscle strength and muscle training after stroke. *Journal of Rehabilitation Medicine* Jan;39(1):14-20

Bohannon RW & Walsh S. (1991). Association of paretic lower extremity muscle strength and standing balance with stair-climbing ability in patients with stroke. *Journal of Stroke and Cerebrovascular Diseases* 1(3): 129-133

Bohannon RW & Walsh S. (1992). Nature, reliability, and predictive value of muscle performance measures in patients with hemiparesis following stroke. *Archives of Physical Medicine and Rehabilitation* Aug;73(8):721-5

Bonita R, Beaglehole R. (1988). Recovery of motor function after stroke. *Stroke* Dec; 19(12): 1497–1500

Cameron D & Bohannon RW. (2000). Criterion validity of lower extremity Motricity Index scores. *Clinical Rehabilitation* Apr;14(2):208-11

Carey, LM. (1995). Somatosensory loss after stroke. *Critical Reviews in Physical & Rehabilitation Medicine* 7:51-91

Carin-Levy G, Greig C, Young A, Lewis S, Hannan J & Mead G. (2006). Longitudinal changes in muscle strength and mass after acute stroke. *Cerebrovasc Dis* 21(3):201-7

Collen FM, Wade DT, Robb GF & Bradshaw CM. (1991). The Rivermead Mobility Index: a further development of the Rivermead Motor Assessment. *International Disability Studies* Apr-Jun;13(2):50-4

Collin C & Wade D. (1990). Assessing motor impairment after stroke: a pilot reliability study. *Journal of Neurology, Neurosurgery, and Psychiatry* Jul;53(7):576-9

Corrigan D & Bohannon RW. (2001). Relationship between knee extension force and stand-up performance in community-dwelling elderly women. *Archives of Physical Medicine and Rehabilitation* Dec;82(12):1666-72

Dattola R, Girlanda P, Vita G, Santoro M, Roberto ML, Toscano A, Venuto C, Baradello A & Messina C. (1993). Muscle rearrangement in patients with hemiparesis after stroke: an electrophysiological and morphological study. *European Neurology* 33(2):109-14

De Deyne PG, Hafer-Macko CE, Ivey FM, Ryan AS & Macko RF. (2004). Muscle molecular phenotype after stroke is associated with gait speed. *Muscle & Nerve* Aug;30(2):209-15

De Haart M, Geurts A, Huidekoper SC, Fasotti L, van Limbeek I. (2004). Recovery of standing balance in post-acute stroke patients: a rehabilitation cohort study. *Archives of Physical Medicine and Rehabilitation* June;85(6):886-95

de Ruiter CJ, Kooistra RD, Paalman MI & de Haan A. (2004). Initial phase of maximal voluntary and electrically stimulated knee extension torque development at different knee angles. *Journal of Applied Physiology* Nov;97(5):1693-701

Demeurisse G, Demol O & Robaye E. (1980). Motor evaluation in vascular hemiplegia. *European Neurology* 19(6), 382-9

Desrosiers J, Malouin F, Richards C, Bourbonnais D, Rochette A, Bravo G. (2003). Comparison of changes in upper and lower extremity impairments and disabilities after stroke. *International Journal of Rehabilitation Research* Jun;26(2):109-16

Dietz V, Ketelsen UP, Berger W & Quintern J. (1986). Motor unit involvement in spastic paresis. Relationship between leg muscle activation and histochemistry. *Journal of Neurological Sciences* Aug;75(1):89-103

Duncan PW, Goldstein lB, Matchar D, Divine GW, Feussner J. (1992). Measurement of motor recovery after stroke. Outcome assessment and sample size requirements. *Stroke* Aug;23:1084–89

Duncan PW, Goldstein LB, Horner RD, Landsman PB, Samsa GP, Matchar DB. (1994). Similar motor recovery of upper and lower extremities after stroke. *Stroke* June;25(6):1181-88

Edstrom L. (1970). Selective changes in the sizes of red and white muscle fibres in upper motor lesions and Parkinsonism. *Journal of Neurological Sciences* Dec;11(6):537-50.

El-Abd MAR, Ibrahim IK. (1994). Impaired afferent control in patients with spastic hemiplegia at different stages of recovery: contribution to gait disorder. *Archives of Physical Medicine and Rehabilitation* Mar;75(3):312-7.

Fugl-Meyer AR, Jaasko L, Leyman I, Olsson S & Steglind S. (1975). The post-stroke hemiplegic patient. 1. a method for evaluation of physical performance. *Scandinavian Journal of Rehabilitation Medicine* 7(1):13-31

Gerrits KH, Beltman MJ, Koppe PA, Konijnenbelt H, Elich PD, de Haan A & Janssen TW. (2009). Isometric muscle function of knee extensors and the relation with functional performance in patients with stroke. *Archives of Physical Medicine and Rehabilitation* Mar;90(3):480-7

Gray CS, French JM, Bates D, Cartlidge NE, James OF, Bates D. (1990). Motor recovery following acute stroke). *Age and Ageing* May;19(3):179-84

Gresham GE, Duncan PW, Stason WB, Adams HP, Adelman AM, Alexander DN, Bishop DS, Diller L, Donaldson NE, Granger CV, Holland AL, Kelly-Hayes M, McDowell FH, Myers L, Phipps MA, Roth EJ, Siebens HC, Tarvin GA, Trombley CA. (1995). *Clinical Practice Guideline Number 16: Post-Stroke Rehabilitation.* Rockville, Md: US Department of Health and Human Services, Public Health Service, Agency for Health Care Policy and Research. AHCPR Publication 95-0662

Hachisuka K, Umezu Y & Ogata H. (1997). Disuse muscle atrophy of lower limbs in hemiplegic patients. *Archives of Physical Medicine and Rehabilitation* Jan;78(1):13-8

Harris ML, Polkey MI, Bath PM & Moxham J. (2001). Quadriceps muscle weakness following acute hemiplegic stroke. *Clinical Rehabilitation* Jun;15(3):274-81

Hendricks HT, van Limbeek J, Geurts AC, Zwarts MJ. (2002). Motor recovery after stroke: a systematic review of the literature. *Archives of Physical Medicine and Rehabilitation* Nov;83(11):1629-37

Holden MK, Gill KM & Magliozzi MR. (1986). Gait assessment for neurologically impaired patients. Standards for outcome assessment. *Physical Therapy* Oct;66(10):1530-9

Holden MK, Gill KM, Magliozzi MR, Nathan J & Piehl-Baker L. (1984). Clinical gait assessment in the neurologically impaired. Reliability and meaningfulness. *Physical Therapy* Jan;64(1):35-40

Horgan NF, Finn AM. (1997). Motor recovery following stroke: a basis for evaluation. *Disability and Rehabilitation* Feb;19(2):64-70

Horstman AM, Beltman MJ, Gerrits KH, Koppe P, Janssen TW, Elich P & de Haan A. (2008). Intrinsic muscle strength and voluntary activation of both lower limbs and functional performance after stroke. *Clinical Physiology and Functional Imaging* Jul;28(4):251-61

Horstman AM, Gerrits KH, Beltman MJ, Koppe PA, Janssen TW & de Haan A. (2010). Intrinsic properties of the knee extensor muscles after subacute stroke. *Archives of Physical Medicine and Rehabilitation* Jan;91(1):123-8

Hubbard IJ, Parsons MW, Neilson C & Carey LM. (2009). Task-specific training: evidence for and translation to clinical practice. *Occupational Therapy International* 16(3-4):175-89

Inaba M, Edberg E, Montgomery J & Gillis MK. (1973). Effectiveness of functional training, active exercise, and resistive exercise for patients with hemiplegia. *Physical Therapy* Jan;53(1):28-35

Johansson BB. (2000). Brain plasticity and stroke rehabilitation. The Willis lecture. *Stroke* Jan;31(1):223–230

Jorgensen HS, Nakayama H, Raaschou HO, Vive-Larsen J, Stoier M & Olsen TS. (1995). Outcome and time course of recovery in stroke. Part II: Time course of recovery. The Copenhagen Stroke Study. *Archives of Physical Medicine and Rehabilitation* May;76(5):406-12

Jorgensen L & Jacobsen BK. (2001). Changes in muscle mass, fat mass, and bone mineral content in the legs after stroke: a 1 year prospective study. *Bone* Jun;28(6):655-9

Kim CM & Eng JJ. (2003). The relationship of lower-extremity muscle torque to locomotor performance in people with stroke. *Physical Therapy* Jan;83(1):49-57

Kim CM, Eng JJ, MacIntyre DL & Dawson AS. (2001). Effects of isokinetic strength training on walking in persons with stroke: a double-blind controlled pilot study. *Journal of Stroke and Cerebrovascular Diseases* Nov-Dec;10(6):265-73

Kong KH, Chua KS, lee J. (2011). Recovery of upper limb dexterity in patients more than 1 year after stroke: frequency, clinical correlates and predictors *NeuroRehabilitation* 28(2):105–11

Kooistra RD, de Ruiter CJ & de Haan A. (2005). Muscle activation and blood flow do not explain the muscle length-dependent variation in quadriceps isometric endurance. *Journal of Applied Physiology* Mar;98(3):810-6

Kwakkel G, Kollen B & Lindeman E. (2004). Understanding the pattern of functional recovery after stroke: Facts and theories. *Restorative Neurology and Neuroscience* 22(3-5):281-99

Lin S. (2005). Motor function and joint position sense in relation to gait performance in chronic stroke patients. *Archives of Physical Medicine and Rehabilitation* Feb;86(2):197-203

Lind K. (1982). A synthesis of studies on stroke rehabilitation. *Journal of Chronic Diseases* Feb;35(2):133-49

Marigold D, Eng J, Tokuno CD, Donnelly CA. (2004). Contribution of muscle strength and integration of afferent input to postural instability in persons with stroke. *Neurorehabilitation and Neural Repair* Dec;18(4):222-9

Mayo NE, Wood-Dauphinee S, Ahmed S, Gordon C, Higgins J, McEwen S, Salbach N. (1999). Disablement following stroke. *Disability and Rehabilitation* May-Jun;21(5-6):258-68

Mercier C & Bourbonnais D. (2004). Relative shoulder flexor and handgrip strength is related to upper limb function after stroke. *Clinical Rehabilitation* Mar;18(2):215-21

Morris SL, Dodd KJ & Morris ME. (2004). Outcomes of progressive resistance strength training following stroke: a systematic review. *Clinical Rehabilitation* Feb;18(1):27-39

Newham DJ & Hsiao SF. (2001). Knee muscle isometric strength, voluntary activation and antagonist co-contraction in the first six months after stroke. *Disability and Rehabilitation* Jun 15;23(9):379-86

Nudo RJ, Wise BM, SiFuentes F, Milliken GW. (1996). Neural substrates for the effects of rehabilitative training on motor recovery after ischemic infarct. *Science* Jun;272(5269):1791–94

Ouellette MM, LeBrasseur NK, Bean JF, Phillips E, Stein J, Frontera WR & Fielding RA. (2004). High-intensity resistance training improves muscle strength, self-reported function, and disability in long-term stroke survivors. *Stroke* Jun;35(6):1404-9

Patel AT, Duncan PW, Lai SM, Studenski S. (2000). The relation between impairments and functional outcome post stroke *Archives of Physical Medicine and Rehabilitation* Oct;81(10):1357-63

Patterson SL, Forrester LW, Rodgers MM, Ryan AS, Ivey FM, Sorkin JD & Macko RF. (2007). Determinants of walking function after stroke: differences by deficit severity. *Archives of Physical Medicine and Rehabilitation* Jan;88(1):115-9

Pijnappels M, Reeves ND, Maganaris CN & van Dieen JH. (2008). Tripping without falling; lower limb strength, a limitation for balance recovery and a target for training in the elderly. *Journal of Electromyography and Kinesiology* Apr;18(2):188-96

Podsiadlo D & Richardson S. (1991). The timed "Up & Go": a test of basic functional mobility for frail elderly persons. *Journal of the American Geriatrics Society* 39, Feb;39(2):142-8

Pohl PS, Duncan P, Perera S, Long J, Liu W, Zhou J & Kautz SA. (2002). Rate of isometric knee extension strength development and walking speed after stroke. *Journal of Rehabilitation Research and Development* Nov-Dec;39(6):651-7

Sanford J, Moreland J, Swanson LR, Stratford PW & Gowland C. (1993). Reliability of the Fugl-Meyer assessment for testing motor performance in patients following stroke. *Physical Therapy* Jul;73(7):447-54

Saunders DH, Greig CA, Mead GE, Young A. (2009) Physical fitness training for stroke patients. *Cochrane Database of Systematic Reviews 2009*, Issue 4. Art. No.: CD003316. DOI: 10.1002/14651858.CD003316.pub3

Scelsi R, Lotta S, Lommi G, Poggi P & Marchetti C. (1984). Hemiplegic atrophy. Morphological findings in the anterior tibial muscle of patients with cerebral vascular accidents. *Acta Neuropathologica* 62(4):324-31

Shepherd RB. (2001). Exercise and training to optimize functional motor performance in stroke: driving neural reorganization? *Neural Plasticity* 8(1-2):121-9

Shield A & Zhou S. (2004). Assessing voluntary muscle activation with the twitch interpolation technique. *Sports Medicine* 2004;34(4):253-67

Shigematsu R, Rantanen T, Saari P, Sakari-Rantala R, Kauppinen M, Sipila S & Heikkinen E. (2006). Motor speed and lower extremity strength as predictors of fall-related bone fractures in elderly individuals. *Aging Clinical and Experimental Research* Aug;18(4):320-4

Smith MT & Baer GD. (1999). Achievement of simple mobility milestones after stroke. *Archives of Physical Medicine and Rehabilitation* Apr;80(4):442-7

Sullivan K, Klassen T & Mulroy S. (2006). Combined task-specific training and strengthening effects on locomotor recovery post-stroke: a case study. *Journal of Neurologic Physical Therapy* Sep;30(3):130-41

Sullivan KJ, Brown DA, Klassen T, Mulroy S, Ge T, Azen SP & Winstein CJ. (2007). Effects of task-specific locomotor and strength training in adults who were ambulatory after stroke: results of the STEPS randomized clinical trial. *Physical Therapy* Dec;87(12):1580-602van Nes IJ, van Kessel ME, Schils F, Fasotti L, Geurts AC & Kwakkel G. (2009). Is visuospatial hemineglect longitudinally associated with postural imbalance in the postacute phase of stroke? *Neurorehabilitation and Neural Repair* Oct;23(8):819-24

Tyson SF, Hanley M, Chillala J, Selley AB, Tallis RC. (2008). Sensory loss in hospital-admitted people with stroke: characteristics, associated factors, and relationship with function. *Neurorehabilitation and Neural Repair* Mar-Apr;22(2):166-72

Verheyden G, Nieuwboer A, De Wit L, Thijs V, Dobbelaere J, Devos H, Severijns D, Vanbeveren S, De Weerdt W. (2008). Time course of trunk, arm, leg, and functional recovery after ischemic stroke. *Neurorehabilitation and Neural Repair* Mar-Apr;22(2):173-9

Wade DT & Hewer RL. (1987). Functional abilities after stroke: measurement, natural history and prognosis. *Journal of Neurology, Neurosurgery and Psychiatry* Feb;50(2):177-82

Winstein CJ, Rose DK, Tan SM, Lewthwaite R, Chui HC & Azen SP. (2004). A randomized controlled comparison of upper-extremity rehabilitation strategies in acute stroke: A pilot study of immediate and long-term outcomes. *Archives of Physical Medicine and Rehabilitation* Apr;85(4):620-8

6

The Hierarchical Status of Mobility Disability Predicts Future IADL Disability: A Longitudinal Study on Ageing in Taiwan

Hui-Ya Chen[1,2], Chih-Jung Yeh[2,3], Ching-Yi Wang[1,2*], Hui-Shen Lin[2,3] and Meng-Chih Lee[2,4]
[1]*Chung Shan Medical University/School of Physical Therapy,*
[2]*Center for Education and Research on Geriatrics and Gerontology,*
[3]*Institute of Public Health,*
[4]*Institute of Medicine,*
Taiwan

1. Introduction

As the older population grows dramatically around the world, it is important that health care providers be able to maintain people with an extended life expectancy in an active stage for as long as possible. Being independent in gross mobility functioning is an indicator of healthy and successful aging (Guralnik and Kaplan, 1989). An effective tool that is easy to use for identifying those at early stage of physical function decline is imperative for achieving this goal.

As people age, a majority of elderly individuals develop physical disability. Such development follows a hierarchical order, starting from mobility, then spreading into instrumental activities of daily living (IADL), and finally ending in basic activities of daily living (BADL) (Pinsky et al., 1987; Barberger-Gateau et al., 1995; Barberger-Gateau et al., 2000). As disability in mobility occurs at an earlier stage of the disablement process, it may be an effective indicator by which to identify older adults in an early stage of physical function decline. Identifying such older adults is imperative in order to provide timely health promotion or early intervention programs.

In the literature, mobility disability has been defined as at least one item requiring help, or being unable to perform independently using two items (climbing stairs and walking on a level surface) (Guralnik et al., 1994; Guralnik et al., 1995; Ostir et al., 1998) or three items (heavy housework, climbing stairs, and walking on a level surface) (Jette and Branch, 1981; Guralnik et al., 1994; Barberger-Gateau et al., 1995; Guralnik et al., 1995; Merrill et al., 1997; Barberger-Gateau et al., 2000; Ble et al., 2005; Yogev-Seligmann et al., 2008) in Rosow's scale (Rosow and Breslau, 1966). Using either two or three items, the disadvantage of a dichotomous mobility disability status is the inability to identify those with an intermediate status (those are becoming disabled, but are not yet disabled and thus require timely intervention).

---

*Corresponding Author

The use of a summed number of tasks labeled as difficult has been proposed as a way to categorize the severity of BADL disability (Hing and Bloom, 1991; Manton et al., 1993). The item-wised hierarchical structure of mobility disability has been investigated only by Wang and colleagues using two items (Wang et al., 2005) in a cross-sectional study. They reported that these hierarchies could identify participants with different physical health and performance levels. Thus the item-wise hierarchy of mobility disability is able to monitor the status of mobility disability and to identify those at the stage of decline.

By using item-wise definitions of mobility hierarchy, previous studies in Taiwan have reported that individuals with more advanced mobility disability are associated with more concurrent dependence in IADL and BADL (Chen et al., 2010; Yeh et al., 2010). We therefore predicted a longitudinal relationship between hierarchical status of mobility disability and IADL disability. However, a literature review reveals that the item-wise hierarchical status of mobility disability for identifying individuals at higher risk of further IADL decline, which often follows the development of mobility disability (Pinsky et al., 1987; Barberger-Gateau et al., 1995; Barberger-Gateau et al., 2000), has not been substantiated. Furthermore, the median age of onset and the required time for 50% of people at different levels of mobility disability to develop IADL disability have not been reported. The required length of time to develop future IADL disability after the onset of each hierarchical mobility disability status is worthwhile to ascertain so that health care providers will be able to estimate how much time they have for early interventions.

Besides the current mobility disability status that might predict future disablement, other risk factors have been reported in the literature, including age, sex, spouse status (Reynolds and Silverstein, 2003), educational level, current working status, cigarette smoking, alcohol consumption, exercise habits (Miller et al., 2000; Sarkisian et al., 2000), number of co-morbidities (Reynolds and Silverstein, 2003), self-rated health (Cornette, 2005), depressive symptoms (Sarkisian et al., 2000; Kazama et al., 2010), and cognition (Reynolds and Silverstein, 2003; Cornette, 2005; Yochim et al., 2008). These will be used, in this study, as covariates to ascertain the significance of mobility disability status in predicting future IADL disablement.

Thus, this study aimed to investigate the predictive validity of a four-level item-wise hierarchical mobility disability status for future IADL disability, using longitudinal data from a national representative sample. The specific purposes were (1) to ascertain the longitudinal relationship between hierarchies of mobility disability and IADL using the hazard ratio of the hierarchical mobility disability status in developing IADL disability across four and eight years of follow up. In order to ascertain the significant contribution of the hierarchical mobility status to IADL disability, we adjusted the potential risk factors that have been reported in the literature; and (2) to report the median age onset and the survival time for 50% of individuals to development of IADL disability (median survival time) in each hierarchical mobility disability stage.

2. Methods

Data were obtained from the 1999, 2003, and 2007 "Survey of Health and Living Status of the Elderly in Taiwan," a population-based longitudinal study with a nationally representative random sample. The sampling was conducted with a three-stage equal probability method. In the first stage, samples were stratified into administrative units; in the second stage, blocks in the selected administrative units were defined as clusters; and in the third stage, two respondents were selected systematically from the register in each block. An elderly cohort of 4,049 individuals aged 60 or older was first interviewed in 1989 and re-interviewed every three to four years until 2007 (response rate = 88.9 - 91.8%). An additional cohort of 2642 individuals aged 50 to 66 was recruited in 1996 and re-interviewed every four years until 2007 (response rate = 81.2 - 92.1%). Full details of the survey have been published elsewhere (Hsu, 2005; Chen et al., 2010).

A total of 4,440 respondents were interviewed in the survey year 1999. For the purposes of our study, we first excluded those who were younger than 60 years old or who did not live in the community, leaving a sample size of 3,465. Another 4 and 47 respondents respectively had incomplete baseline data in mobility and other variables, such as education attainment, work status, spouse status, health lifestyle, disease status, self-rated health, BADL, and IADL, and were also excluded, further reducing the sample size to 3,414. In order to determine the risk of developing future IADL disability of each mobility disability group, we further excluded 977 individuals who already had IADL disability at baseline, leaving 2,437. Furthermore, we excluded 25 individuals due to loss of contact for follow-up and 285 individuals due to death before contributing any follow-up data on IADL in the years of 2003 and 2007. As a result, 2,127 community-dwelling older adults who had complete baseline data, were free of IADL disability at baseline, and contributed follow-up data at least once remained for further survival analysis of median age onset and the median survival time of IADL disability for each hierarchical status of mobility disability.

For Cox regression, we used the extended-model approach for covariate adjustment: Model 1 = without adjustment; Model 2 = variables in Model 1 + demographics (age, sex, education, work, and spouse status); Model 3 = variables in Models 1 & 2 + health behaviors (smoking, alcohol, and exercise); Model 4 = variables in Models 1 & 2 & 3 + health status (number of co-morbidities, self-rated health, the Center for Epidemiologic Studies Depression (CESD), and Short Portable Mental Status Questionnaire (SPMSQ)). Data on 2,127 (at eight-year follow-up) and 2,073 (at four-year follow-up, with an additional 54 samples excluded due to loss of contact for follow-up in 2003) individuals were entered into Model 1. The amount of data entered into Model 4, however, decreased dramatically because participants younger than 65 were not interviewed for their cognitive function in the survey. In total, data on cognitive function (SPMSQ) were missing for 574 (eight-year follow-up) and 557 (four-year follow-up) individuals, and data on the CESD scale were missing for 8 individuals. As a result, we excluded the data from 582 (eight-year follow-up) and 565 (four-year follow-up) individuals when running Model Four in Cox regression.

2.1 Measurements

2.1.1 Four-level hierarchy of mobility disability

This study extracted from the survey questionnaire three variables assessing gross mobility: heavy housework, climbing up 2 to 3 floors, and walking 200 to 300 m. Those reporting no difficulty in performing all three items were in the "mobility able" group, whereas those reporting difficulty performing only one item were categorized as "1 item disabled". Those reporting difficulty in any two of the three items or in all three items were treated as "2 items disabled" and "3 items disabled", respectively.

2.1.2 IADL disability status

There were five items in the instrumental activities of daily living (IADL) domain (shopping, finance, transportation, light housework, and telephone). Older adults were classified as having IADL disability if they reported any degree of difficulty or inability to perform on at least one item.

2.1.3 Covariates in Cox regressions

Covariates were included in the Cox regression models according to their values in 1999. Age was categorical data, whereas sex, current working status, smoking habit, and alcohol ingestion were dichotomous data. Education was recorded as illiteracy or no formal education, elementary school, primary or senior high school, and college or beyond. Spouse status was recorded as either living with spouse (married or living together) or living without spouse (never married, divorced, separated, or widowed).

The exercise habit was divided into inactive (less than three times a week) and active (at least three times a week). Self-rated health was divided into healthier and worsening. The number of co-morbidities was counted from the list of hypertension, diabetes, cardiac disease, stroke, cancer, and arthritis. Cognitive function was measured with the modified Taiwan version of SPMSQ using nine items (range 0-9), correct answers were coded 1, whereas errors were coded 0, thus, higher SPMSQ score means better cognition performance, individuals were categorized as having normal (6 and above) or abnormal (5 and below) cognitive function (Yen et al., 2010). Symptoms of depression were assessed with the CESD, on which each of the 10 items is scored from 0 to 3. Individuals were categorized as not having (9 and below) or having (10 and above) depressive symptoms.

2.2 Statistical analysis

The group means difference among the four hierarchical mobility disability groups was determined by analysis of variance (ANOVA) for the continuous variables and chi-square test for discrete variables. Median age difference among the four groups were investigated by Brown-Mood test. The group comparison on the depression score among the four groups was determined by using the ANOVA on the log transformed CESD score. Cox proportional hazard regression analysis was used to determine if the hierarchical mobility disability stage was a significant predictor of future IADL disability four years later (in 2003) and eight years later (in 2007) and to report its hazard ratio.

The median age onset of IADL disability of each hierarchical mobility disability group across eight years of follow up was determined by survival analysis. The survival time for 50% of participants in each hierarchical status of mobility disability to develop IADL disability (the median survival time) was determined for the whole group and separately for men and women.

3. Results

The demographic and health related information of our participants in the hierarchical mobility disability groups are summarized in Table 1. All variables showed significant differences among the four hierarchical mobility disability groups and were used as covariates in the following Cox regression analysis. The "mobility able" group was younger; had larger percentages of men; had higher educational levels, larger percentages currently working, and spouses; smoked, drank alcohol, and exercised; and had a lower number of co-morbidities, a better perceived health status, better cognition, and lower depression symptom scores.

	Mobility Able (n=1531)	1 Item Disabled (n=359)	2 Items Disabled (n=168)	3 Items Disabled (n=69)
Age (yrs) [¥, a]	70 (64, 73)	73 (67, 77)	72 (67.5, 75)	71 (68, 75)
Sex (n, %) [a, e]				
Men	997 (65.1%)	173 (49.2%)	58 (34.5%)	29 (42.0%)
Women	534 (34.9%)	186 (51.8%)	110 (65.5%)	40 (58.0%)
Educational level (n, %) [a]				
Illiterate	332 (21.7%)	116 (32.3%)	68 (40.5%)	31 (44.9%)
Elementary school	761 (49.6%)	163 (45.4%)	82 (48.8%)	31 (44.9%)
Junior or senior high school	324 (21.2%)	61 (17.0%)	15 (8.9%)	6 (8.7%)
Above college	114 (7.5%)	19 (5.3%)	3 (1.8%)	1 (1.5%)
Work status (missing data, n=7) (n, %)[b, c]				
No	1153 (75.3%)	320 (89.1%)	156 (92.9%)	61 (88.4%)
Yes	378 (24.7%)	39 (10.9%)	12 (7.1%)	8 (11.6%)
Spouse status (missing data, n=1) (n, %)[b, c]				
No	410 (26.8%)	135 (37.6%)	61 (36.3%)	27 (39.1%)
Yes	1121 (73.2%)	224 (62.4%)	107 (63.7%)	42 (60.9%)
Cigarette smoking (n, %) [b, c]				
No	1073 (70.1%)	289 (80.5%)	139 (82.7%)	56 (81.2%)
Yes	458 (29.9%)	70 (19.5%)	29 (17.3%)	13 (18.8%)
Alcohol consumption (n, %) [a]				
No	1049 (68.5%)	290 (80.8%)	141 (83.9%)	61 (88.4%)
Yes	482 (31.5%)	69 (19.2%)	27 (16.1%)	8 (11.6%)
Exercise (n, %)*, [c]				
No	539 (35.2%)	136 (37.9%)	75 (44.6%)	36 (52.2%)
Yes	992 (64.8%)	223 (62.1%)	93 (55.4%)	33 (47.8%)
Number of co-morbidities [f] (hypertension, DM, cardiac disease, stroke, cancer, arthritis)	0.7 ± 0.9	1.1 ± 1.0	1.3 ± 1.1	1.5 ± 1.2
Self Perceived Health Status (n, %)[a, d]				
Worse	227 (14.8%)	128 (35.6%)	79 (47.0%)	41 (59.4%)
Healthier	1304 (85.2%)	231 (64.4%)	89 (53.0%)	28 (40.6%)
Cognition_SPMSQ [f]	8.6 ± 0.8 (n=1081)	8.3 ± 1.1 (n=280)	8.1 ± 1.3 (n=139)	8.0 ± 1.3 (n=53)
Depression_CESD-10 [a]	3.4 ± 4.3 (n=1504)	5.9 ± 5.7 (n=341)	7.5 ± 6.1 (n=166)	8.6 ± 7.0 (n=64)

[¥]: median (q1,q3), [a] significant differences were found between "mobility able group and all other (1 item, 2 items, and 3 items) disabled" groups; [b] significant differences were found between "mobility able and 2 items disabled"; [c] significant differences were found between "mobility able and 3 items disabled" group; [d] significant differences was found between "1 item disabled and 3 items disabled groups"; [e] significant differences was found between "1 item disabled and 2 items disabled groups"; [f] no statistical significance between item 2 and item 3.

Table 1. Demographic and health-related information at baseline (year of 1999) (n=2127).

Tables 2 and 3 show the results of the Cox regression models, with significant effects of the hierarchy of mobility on developing IADL disability. As shown in Table 2, the unadjusted hazard ratios for developing IADL disability after four years, with "mobility able" as the reference group, were as follows: 2.15 for "1 item disabled", 3.09 for "2 items disabled", and 3.63 for "3 items disabled". After adjustment for potential risk factors, the hierarchical structure of hazard ratios of the four-level mobility status remained the same, though diminished in value (1.55, 1.85, and 2.19), yet they were still the strongest among the significant risk factors.

	Model 1	Model 2	Model 3	Model 4
Mobility Able	1	1	1	1
1 Item Disabled	2.15 (1.75-2.68)***	1.59(1.27-2.00)***	1.57 (1.25-1.98)**	1.55 (1.21-1.99)**
2 Items Disabled	3.09 (2.40-3.98)***	2.17 (1.67-2.83)**	2.14 (1.64-2.79)***	1.85 (1.37-2.50)***
3 Items Disabled	3.63 (2.59-5.10)***	2.61 (1.85-3.69)**	2.48 (1.74-3.52)***	2.19 (1.46-3.28)**
Age				
60-65 years		1	1	1
65-70 years		1.58 (1.09-2.29)*	1.60 (1.10-2.33)*	0.89 (0.12-6.61)
70-75 years		2.14 (1.55-2.96)**	2.19 (1.58-3.03)***	1.13 (0.15-8.29)
Over 75 years		3.24 (2.33-4.49)**	3.30 (2.37-4.59)***	1.80 (0.25-13.20)
Sex				
Men vs. Women		0.80 (0.65-0.98)*	0.79 (0.63-1.00)*	0.80 (0.62-1.03)
Educational level				
Illiterate		1	1	1
Elementary school		0.71 (0.58-0.88)**	0.72 (0.59-0.90)**	0.78 (0.62-0.99)*
Junior or senior school		0.63 (0.46-0.85)**	0.65 (0.48-0.88)**	0.72 (0.52-0.99)*
College and above		0.77 (0.43-1.07)	0.73 (0.46-1.17)	0.80 (0.49-1.31)
Work status				
Yes vs. No		0.69 (0.50-0.95) *	0.68 (0.50-0.94)*	0.76 (0.53-1.09)
Spouse status				
Yes vs. No		0.97 (0.79-1.18)	0.96 (0.79-1.17)	1.03 (0.83-1.28)
Cigarette smoking				
Yes vs. No			1.23 (0.96-1.57)	1.30 (1.00-1.69)
Alcohol consumption				
Yes vs. No			0.77 (0.60-1.00)*	0.75 (0.57-0.99)*
Exercise				
Yes vs. No			0.89 (0.73-1.08)	0.96 (0.78-1.18)
No. of co-morbidities				1.12 (1.02-1.24)*
Self rated health				
Good vs. Poor				1.03 (0.82-1.29)
SPMSQ				1.39 (0.90-2.17)
CESD-10				1.31 (1.03-1.67)*

*** <0.0001, ** <0.01, *<0.05

Table 2. Hazard ratio of each hierarchical mobility disability group to develop IADL disability across 4 years follow-up (years of 1999-2003) (n=2073).

In the final model, significant risk factors for developing IADL disability were mobility disability stage, educational level, alcohol consumption, number of co-morbidities, and depression symptom score. It should be noted that age, sex, and working status were significant risk factors in Models 2 & 3, but became insignificant in the final Model 4, with more covariates relating to health status.

Similar to those from the four-year follow-up data, the hazard ratios for developing IADL disability after eight years were also hierarchical, but they had smaller values: 1.96, 2.64, and 2.88 for the groups of "1 item disabled", "2 items disabled", and "3 items disabled", respectively (Table 3). The final model in the eight-year follow-up, when compared to the four-year follow-up data, had more covariates: sex, educational level, cigarette smoking, number of co-morbidities, and cognition.

The median age at onset for "mobility able", "1 item disabled", 2 items disabled", and "3 items disabled" group was 82, 80, 77, and 76 years of age, respectively. The median survival time is reported for each hierarchical stage of mobility disability and as follows: greater than 8 years for "mobility able", 6 years for "1 item disabled", 6 years for "2 items disabled", and 2 years for "3 items disabled" (Table 4). Inspection of the data in the four mobility disability groups revealed that it took longer period for men than for women to develop IADL disability.

Mobility disability at baseline	N	Median survival time (years)
Men		
Mobility Able	997	– (6, –)
1 Item Disabled	173	6 (2, –)
2 Items Disabled	58	6 (2, –)
3 Items Disabled	29	2 (2, 7)
Women		
Mobility Able	534	7 (4, –)
1 Item Disabled	186	6 (2, –)
2 Items Disabled	110	2 (2, 6)
3 Items Disabled	40	2 (2, –)
All		
Mobility Able	1531	8 (6, –)
1 Item Disabled	359	6 (2, –)
2 Items Disabled	168	4 (2, –)
3 Items Disabled	69	2 (2, –)

–: not defined

Table 3. The median survival time for each hierarchical status of mobility disability (8 years of follow up, 1999-2007) (n=2127).

4. Discussion

The purposes of this study were to ascertain the longitudinal relationship of developing the mobility disability and IADL disability and to report the hazard ratio, the median age onset, and the median survival time to the onset of IADL disability in each hierarchical stage of mobility disability for use in the development of early intervention programs. In this study, we defined a four-level hierarchy of disability severity in the mobility domain by the summed number of items labeled as difficult among three items: heavy housework, climbing stairs, and walking on a level surface. Our results indicate that the hierarchy of mobility disability used in this study can significantly identify people with different demographics, health behaviors, and health status. Furthermore, this hierarchical mobility status also has a hierarchical structure in terms of the hazard ratio, the median age onset, and the median survival time to development of IADL disability.

Assessing a hierarchy of mobility disability based on the numbers of items disabled can discriminate between older adults with different levels of physical performance (Wang et al., 2005). The results of this study further substantiate the predictive validity of this hierarchy of mobility disability for future IADL disability at four years and eight years later. Individuals with more severe levels of mobility disability were at greater risk of developing IADL disability, even after adjusting for other risk factors of demographics, health behaviors, and health status. From the magnitude of hazard ratio in the final Cox model, it could be seen that the level of mobility disability appeared to be the strongest predictor of future IADL disability. To the best of our knowledge, this is the first study to examine the predictive validity of the item-wise hierarchy of mobility disability for future IADL disability based on longitudinal follow up on a nationally representative sample of the Taiwanese community-dwelling elderly.

Consistent with previous studies, demographics such as age, sex, and working status were significant risk factors in the initial Cox models (Jette & Branch, 1981; Pinsky et al., 1987; Guralnik & Kaplan, 1989), but they became insignificant in the final model due to the addition of covariates related to health status. Health status, namely number of co-morbidities, cognition, and depression symptom score, were significant risk factors in the final model. However, from the perspective of health promotion, demographics such as age and gender are non-modifiable and hence are not the focus of discussion in this study. Education and the health behaviors that were found to be significant risk factors of IADL disability in the current study, such as health status, alcohol consumption, and cigarette smoking, are in agreement with the literature (Jette & Branch, 1981; Pinsky et al., 1987; Guralnik & Kaplan, 1989) and are valuable in guiding health promotion policy or programs for people at younger ages. For example, policy for extending the years for obligatory education could help people get higher education, and that might in turn lead to better socioeconomic status and policy for health education for the publics could facilitate better health behaviors. Heightened socioeconomic status and better health behaviors could lessen the numbers of comorbidities people will develop during the process of ageing and decrease the negative impact that comorbidities might have on cognitive function and emotional health.

Surprisingly, habitual exercise was not significant in either the four or eight-year follow-up, and we propose two possibilities for this insignificance. First, our dichotomous cutting point was based on frequency of exercise per week, which did not consider exercise intensity and may fail to reflect the health benefits of exercises. Second, general exercise may be insufficient for people who already have some mobility disability, and specific training for specific impairments may be necessary, such as intervention for joint range of motion and lower leg eccentric contraction to improve the ability to climb stairs. Previous research has suggested that heavy housework requires more muscle power, whole-body strength, balance and coordination, while climbing stairs and walking on a level surface require standing balance and lower extremity strength and velocity (Bean et al., 2008; Chen et al., 2010). Early intervention for mobility performance and stability needs to take into consideration these task-specific impairments.

The results of this study confirm the time window that health care providers have in order to reverse mobility disability and to prevent IADL disability. Our findings suggest that people with two or more items disabled in mobility develop IADL disability in 2-4 years, whereas people with one or less items disabled in mobility develop IADL disability in 6 years or longer. The survival analyses further suggested that men and women have different disablement patterns. In general, the interval for 50% of participants to develop IADL disability (median survival time) was shorter for women than that for men. Therefore, in health promotion or early intervention, the different time windows for men and women should be taken into consideration.

In this Taiwan Longitudinal Study on Ageing (TLSA) dataset, individuals were followed up every four year. The data of the year of 1999, 2003, and 2007 were used in the current study that included two follow-ups at 4 years and 8 years later. The 3rd quartile was not reported from the statistics output of the survival analysis, it is probably because the maximal follow up duration was 8-year and by that time not yet 75% of the individuals developed that certain hierarchical disability level. This study was also limited by the long interval of follow up (every four years). However, a shorter follow-up period consumes more resources. The need for a balance between the large cost and the additional information that could be gathered by a shorter follow-up period needs to be carefully considered. In addition, the population in our study was free of IADL disability at baseline, with 977 individuals excluded due to initial IADL disability. Our results should not be generalized to people who have both mobility and IADL disability. Furthermore, mobility disability is a changing condition, but our prediction of future IADL disability was based only on baseline mobility status.

5. Conclusion

The hierarchical status of mobility disability is the strongest predictor of IADL disability even after adjustments for the significant risk factors of demographics, health behaviors, and health status. Very different results of IADL disability development were found between the groups with two or more items disabled and those with one or less items disabled in mobility, which provides support for the value of hierarchical stages of mobility categorization, as opposed to the previous dichotomous definition, with any one item disabled.

People who have more disabled mobility items but are free of IADL disability initially are at higher risk of developing IADL disability than those with one or less item disabled, and the time to development is only 2-4 years. We suggest that health care providers focus on people who have two or more items disabled in mobility and that they intervene within the time window of 2-4 years in order to reverse mobility disability or to prevent IADL disability, both of which are situated in the earlier stages of the disablement process.

6. Acknowledgment

We thank the Population and Health Research Center, Bureau of Health Promotion, Department of Health, Taiwan, Republic of China, for providing the data.

7. References

Barberger-Gateau, P.; Nejjari, C.; Tessier, J. F. & Dartigues, J. F. (1995). Assessment of disability and handicap associated with dyspnoea in elderly subjects. *Disability and Rehabilitation* Vol. 17, No. 2, (Feb-Mar, 1999), 83-89, ISSN 0963-8288.

Barberger-Gateau, P.; Rainville, C.; Letenneur, L. & Dartigues, J. F. (2000). A hierarchical model of domains of disablement in the elderly: a longitudinal approach. *Disability and Rehabilitation* Vol. 22, No. 7, (2000), 308-317, ISSN 0963-8288.

Bean, J. F.; Kiely, D. K.; LaRose, S. & Leveille, S. G. (2008). Which impairments are most associated with high mobility performance in older adults? Implications for a rehabilitation prescription. *Archives of Physical Medicine and Rehabilitation* Vol. 89, (December 2008), 2278-2284. ISSN 1532-821X.

Ble, A.; Volpato, S.; Zuliani, G.; Guralnik, J. M.; Bandinelli, S.; Lauretani, F.; Bartali, B.; Maraldi, C.; Fellin, R. & Ferrucci, L. (2005). Executive function correlates with walking speed in older persons: the InCHIANTI study. *Journal of the American Geriatrics Society* Vol. 53, No. 3, (March, 2005), 410-415, ISSN 0002-8614.

Chen, H. Y.; Wang, C. Y.; Lee, M. Y.; Tang, P. F.; Chu, Y. S. & Suen, M. W. (2010). A hierarchical categorisation of tasks in mobility disability. *Disability and Rehabilitation* Vol. 32, No. 19, (2010), 1586-1593, ISSN 0963-8288.

Cornette, P.; Swine, C.; Malhomme, B.; Gillet, J. B.; Meert, P. & D'Hoore, W. (2005). Early evaluation of the risk of functional decline following hospitalization of older patients: development of a predictive tool. *European Journal of Public Health* Vol. 16, No. 2, (September 2005), 203-208.

Guralnik, J. M. & Kaplan, G. A. (1989). Predictors of healthy aging: prospective evidence from the Alameda County study. *American Journal of Public Health* Vol. 79, No. 6, (June 1989), 703-708, ISSN 1541-0048.

Guralnik, J. M.; Simonsick, E. M.; Ferrucci, L.; Glynn, R. J.; Berkman, L. F.; Blazer, D. G.; Scherr, P. A. & Wallace, R. B. (1994). A short physical performance battery assessing lower extremity function: association with self-reported disability and prediction of mortality and nursing home admission. *Journal of Gerontology* Vol. 49, No. 2, (March 1994), M85-M94, ISSN 0022-1422.

Guralnik, J. M.; Ferrucci, L.; Simonsick, E. M.; Salive, M. E. & Wallace, R. B. (1995). Lower-extremity function in persons over the age of 70 years as a predictor of subsequent disability. *The New England Journal of Medicine* Vol. 332, No. 9, (March, 1995), 556-561, ISSN 1533-4406.

Hing, E. & Bloom, B. (1991). Long-term care for the functionally dependent elderly. *American Journal of Public Health* Vol. 81, No. 2, (Feburary 1991), 223-225. ISSN 0090-0036.

Hsu, H. C. Gender disparity of successful aging in Taiwan. *Women & Health* Vol. 42, No. 1, (2005), 1-21, ISSN 0363-0242.

Jette, A. M. & Branch, L. G. (1981). The Framingham Disability Study: II. Physical disability among the aging. *American Journal of Public Health* Vol. 71, No. 11, (November 1981), 1211-1216, ISSN 0090-0036.

Kazama, M.; Kondo, N.; Suzuki, K.; Minai, J.; Imai, H. & Yamagata, Z. (2010). Early impact of depression symptoms on the decline in activities of daily living among older Japanese: Y-HALE cohort study. *Environmental Health and Preventive Medicine* Vol. 16, No. 3, (November, 2010), 196-201, ISSN 1342-078X.

Manton, K. G.; Corder, L. S. & Stallard, E. (1993). Estimates of change in chronic disability and institutional incidence and prevalence rates in the U.S. elderly population from the 1982, 1984, and 1989 National Long Term Care Survey. *Journal of Gerontology* Vol. 48, No. 4, (1993), S153-S166, ISSN 0022-1422.

Merrill, S. S.; Seeman, T. E.; Kasl, S. V. & Berkman, L. F. (1997). Gender differences in the comparison of self-reported disability and performance measures. *The Journals of Gerontology. Series A, Biological Sciences and Medical Sciences* Vol. 52, No. 1, (1997), M19-M26, ISSN 1079-5006.

Miller, M. E.; Rejeski, W. J.; Reboussin, B. A.; Ten Have, T. R. & Ettinger, W. H. (2000). Physical activity, functional limitations, and disability in older adults. *Journal of the American Geriatrics Society* Vol. 48, No. 10, (October 2000), 1264-1272, ISSN 0002-8614.

Ostir, G. V.; Markides, K. S.; Black, S. A. & Goodwin, J. S. (1998). Lower body functioning as a predictor of subsequent disability among older Mexican Americans. *The Journals of Gerontology. Series A, Biological Sciences and Medical Sciences* Vol. 53, No. 6, (1998), M491-M495, ISSN 1079-5006.

Pinsky, J. L.; Leaverton, P. E. & Stokes, J. 3rd. (1987). Predictors of good function: the Framingham Study. *Journal of chronic diseases* Vol. 40, Suppl 1, (1987), 159S-167S, ISSN 0021-9681.

Reynolds, S. L. & Silverstein, M. (2003). Observing the onset of disability in older adults. *Social Science and Medicine* Vol. 57, No. 10, (November 2003), 1875-1889, ISSN 0277-9536.

Rosow, I. & Breslau, N. (1966). A Guttman health scale for the aged. *Journal of Gerontology* Vol. 21, No. 4, (October 1966), 556-559, ISSN 0022-1422.

Sarkisian, C. A.; Liu, H.; Gutierrez, P. R.; Seeley, D. G. & Cummings, S. R. (2000). Modifiable risk factors predict functional decline among older women: a prospectively validated clinical prediction tool. The Study of Osteoporotic Fractures Research Group. *Journal of the American Geriatrics Society* Vol. 48, No. 2, (Feburary 2000), 170-178, ISSN 0002-8614.

Yeh, T. T., Wang, C. Y.; Lin, C. F. & Chen, H. Y. (2010). The hierarchical relationship between mobility limitation and ADL disability in older Taiwanese persons. *Formosan Journal of Physical Therapy* Vol. 35, (March 2010), 1-7.

Yochim, B. P.; Lequerica, A.; MacNeil, S. E. & Lichtenberg, P. A. (2008). Cognitive initiation and depression as predictors of future instrumental activities of daily living among older medical rehabilitation patients. *Journal of Clinical and Experimental Neuropsychology* Vol. 30, No. 2, (January 2008), 236-244, ISSN 1380-3395.

Yogev-Seligmann, G.; Hausdorff, J. M. & Giladi, N. (2008). The role of executive function and attention in gait. *Movement Disorders* Vol. 23, No. 3, (February 2008), 329-342, ISSN 0885-3185.

Wang, C. Y.; Olson, S. L.; Gleeson, P. & Protas, E. J. (2005). Physical performance tests to evaluate mobility disability in community-dwelling elders. *Journal of Aging and Physical Activity* Vol. 13, No. 2, (April 2005), 184-197, ISSN 1063-8652.